Adele Gl

INTERMITTENT FASTING

COOKBOOK 2021:

Delicious Recipes To Lose Weight, Stay Healthy
With Intermittent Fasting

Table of Contents

INTRODUCTION 8

CHAPTER 1: THE KETO DIET PLAN FOR INTERMITTENT FASTING 12

MACRO GUIDELINES 15

CALORIE COUNTING VERSUS MICROS... 15

FOODS INCLUDED IN THE INTERMITTENT FASTING PLAN 16

Fresh Vegetables...16

Fresh Fruits...19

Excellent Spices...20

Acceptable Sweeteners...22

Beverage Options 22

Include Healthy Fats & Oils 23

Other Monounsaturated & Saturated Fats 24

Other Choices for the Ketogenic Plan..25

Include These Cold Items..25

CHAPTER 2: HOW TO GET STARTED ON THE 16/8 PLAN........................26

HOW TO BEGIN 26

AVOID THESE FOOD ITEMS... 28

CHAPTER 3: BREAKFAST FAVORITES 32

1.   Almond Coconut Egg Wraps...32

2.   Almonds & Chips Breakfast Cereal 34

3.   Almost McGriddle Casserole...35

4.   Bacon Hash..37

5.   Bagels & Cheese...39

6.   Belgian Style Waffles 41

7.   Biscuits & Gravy 42

8.   Blueberry Flaxseed Muffins 44

9.   Blueberry Ricotta Pancakes 46

10. Chocolate Loaf..48

11. Cinnamon Raisin Bagels..50

12. Classic Bacon & Eggs...52

13. Cocoa Waffles..54

CHAPTER 4: LUNCHTIME OPTIONS..56

14. Bread Twists for the Salad...56

15   Caprese Salad...58

16. Chicken BLT Salad 60

17. Chicken, Feta, & Kiwi Salad 62

18.   Chicken-Pecan Salad & Cucumber Bites 63
19.   Cobb Salad 65
20.   Egg Salad 67
21.   Greek Salad 69
SOUP CHOICES 71
22.   Broccoli Curry Soup 71
23.   Chicken Chowder – Crockpot 73
SEAFOOD 75
24.   Alfredo Shrimp 75
25.   Avocado & Salmon Omelet Wrap 77
OTHER DELICIOUS LUNCHTIME CHOICES 79
26.   Buffalo Cauliflower Bites 79
27.   Chinese Sauce Fried Rice 81

CHAPTER 5: TASTY DINNER CHOICES 83
POULTRY 83
28.   Buffalo Chicken Burgers 83
29.   Chicken & Asparagus 85
PORK 87
30.   BBQ Pork Loin 87
31.   Carnitas – Crockpot 89
32.   Crack Slaw – Pork Egg Roll in a Bowl 91
FISH SEAFOOD OPTIONS 93
33.   Baked Tilapia With Cherry Tomatoes 93
34.   Chili Lime Cod 95
BEEF OPTIONS 97
35.   Bacon Cheeseburger 97
36.   Barbacoa Beef – Kitchen robot 99
37.   BBQ Flank Steak 101
38.   Cheeseburger Calzones 103
39.   Enchilada 105

CHAPTER 6: SNACKTIME TREATS 108
40.   Arancini – 5-Cheese Bacon & Cauliflower Bites 108
41.   BBQ Chicken Pizza 111
42.   Chicken Nuggets 113
43.   Chicken Salad Deviled Eggs 115
44.   Delicious Grilled Cheese Sandwiches 117
SWEET SNACKS 119
45.   Cinnamon Vanilla Protein Bites 119

CHAPTER 7: DESSERT FAVORITES 122
   46.   *Almond & Coconut Cake* 122
   47.   *Brownie Mug Cake – Kitchen robot* 124
   48.   *Cheesecake Pudding* 126
   49.   *Chocolate Chip Cookie Cheesecake Bars* 128
   50.   *Chocolate-Filled Peanut Butter Cookies* 131
   51.   *Chocolate Mini Cakes* 133
   52.   *Coconut-Almond Bars – Kitchen robot* 135
   53.   *Creamy Lime Pie* 137
   54.   *5-Minute Peanut Butter Mousse* 139
   55.   *Keto Magic Bars* 141

CHAPTER 8: 21-DAY SPECIAL MEAL PLAN FOR BUSY PEOPLE 144

CHAPTER 9: TIPS & TRICKS TO CONTROL HUNGER & AVOID MISTAKES 152
  HOW TO MAINTAIN FAT LOSS 152
  RECOGNIZE YOUR CRAVINGS 156
  EAT HEALTHIER SNACKS DURING YOUR EATING WINDOW 157
  BE SURE THE PLAN IS FOR YOU—AVOID MISTAKES 159
  OTHER INTERMITTENT DIETING SUGGESTIONS 160
  ALWAYS CHECK YOUR MEDICATIONS FOR COMPATIBILITY 162
  KNOW-HOW: TEST FOR KETOSIS ACTIVITY 163

CONCLUSION 166

INDEX FOR THE RECIPES: 170

Introduction

Congratulations on purchasing your copy of *Intermittent Fasting*, and thank you for doing so. The following pages will provide you with the groundwork that will be essential for success using the ketogenic diet plan. Before you begin the journey to ketosis, here is a bit of insight on how the diet plan was discovered.

During the era of the 1920s and 1930s, the ketogenic diet was prevalent for its role in epilepsy therapy treatments. The diet plan provided a method other than the uncharacteristic techniques of fasting, which were popular in the treatment plan.

During the 1940s, the process was abandoned because of new therapies for seizures. However, approximately 20 to 30% of the epileptic cases failed to reach control of the epileptic seizures. With that failure, the Keto Diet was reintroduced as a management technique.

The Charlie Foundation was founded by the family of Charlie

Abraham in 1994 after his recovery from seizures and other health issues he suffered daily. Charlie, as a youngster, was placed on the diet and continued to use it for five years. As of 2016, he is still functioning successfully without the seizure episodes and is furthering his education as a college student.

The Charlie Foundation appointed a panel of dietitians and neurologists to form an agreement in the form of a statement in 2006. It was written as an approval of the diet, and it stated which cases it would be considered for use. It is noted that the plan is especially recommended for children.

You will be learning the best of two plans when you use the intermittent fasting techniques, specifically the 16/8 plan. Intermittent fasting has grown in popularity in recent years since it has the ability to endorse higher rates of nutrient absorption in the meals you eat.

The plan has also grown in popularity because it doesn't require adherents to change the types of foods radically you are eating or even alter drastically the number of calories you consume in each 24-hour time frame. In fact, the most common type of intermittent fasting is to eat two substantial meals in a day instead of the usual three.

You have so many choices for the intermittent fasting process by using only the ketogenic diet techniques.

This makes the intermittent fasting diet plan an ideal choice for those who find they have difficulty sticking to more strict diet plans, as it only requires changing one habit, which is the number of meals instead of many habits all at once. It's simple enough to manage successfully over a prolonged period while at the same time being efficient enough to provide the type of results that can keep motivation levels high once the novelty of the new way of eating begins to fade.

The secret to intermittent fasting's accomplishment is the simple fact that the body works contrarily in a fasting status versus a fed state, which is when your body actively digests and absorbs food. This process begins some five minutes after you have finished putting food into your body and can last anywhere from three to five hours, depending on how complicated the food is for your body to digest.

While in the fed state, your body is actively producing insulin, which, in turn, makes it harder to burn fat properly. The period after digestion has occurred; the insulin levels start dropping back toward normal. This process can take (in the neighborhood) from 8 to 12 hours, which is the buffer between the fed and fasted state. Once your insulin levels return to normal, the fasted state begins, and this is the period where your body can process fat most effectively. Sadly, many people never reach the point where they can burn fat most efficiently, as they rarely go eight hours, much less twelve hours from some caloric consumption.

These are several celebrities who affirm that the intermittent fasting works.

Nicole Kidman abides the eight-hour fasting rule and sticks with the veggies and proteins as her guidelines for healthier eating. Justin Theroux used intermittent fasting between 7 in the morning until 7 in the evening. It is a bit more of an eating window, but you need to start somewhere. Choose the 16/8 plan and see how it works for you!

CHAPTER 1:

The Keto Diet Plan for Intermittent Fasting

The keto diet will set up your body to deplete the stored glucose. Once that is accomplished, your body will focus on diminishing the stored fat we have saved as fuel. The new technique will begin with 5% for carbs, 75% fats, and 20% for protein daily. Many people don't understand that counting calories don't matter at this point since it is just used as a baseline. Your body doesn't need glucose, which causes these 2 stages:

- *The Stage of Glycogenesis:* The excess of glucose converts itself into glycogen, which is stored in the muscles and liver. Research indicates that only about half of your energy used daily can be saved as glycogen.

- *The Stage of Lipogenesis:* If there is an adequate supply of glycogen in your liver and muscles, any excess is converted to fat and stored.

Your body will have no more food (much like when you are sleeping), making your body burn the fat to create ketones. Once the ketones break down the fats, which generate fatty acids, they will burn-off in the liver through beta-oxidation. Thus, when you no longer have a supply of glycogen or glucose, ketosis begins, and the consumed/stored fat will be used as energy. The Internet provides you with a keto calculator at "keto-calculator.ankerl.com." Begin your process by making a habit of checking your levels when you want to know what essentials your body needs during the course of your dieting plan. You will document your personal information, such as height and weight. The Internet calculator will provide you with essential math.

When the glycerol and fatty acid molecules are released, the ketogenesis process begins, and acetoacetate is produced. The Acetoacetate is converted to two types of ketone units:

- *Acetone:* This is mostly excreted as waste but can also be metabolized into glucose. This is the reason individuals on a ketogenic diet will experience a distinctive smelly breath.
- *Beta-hydroxybutyrate or BHB:* Your muscles will convert the acetoacetate into BHB, which will fuel your

brain after you have been on the keto diet for a short time.

You will discover how flexible the ketogenic methods are when coupled with the intermittent fasting techniques. You will lose weight differently with each method, and other people may not have the same goals as you.

For now, as a beginner, you will begin by using the first method, as shown below. This is an important step; you must decide how you want to proceed with your diet plan. It is always best to discuss this essential step with your physician. These are the four methods, for you to understand the different levels of the keto diet plan better:

Keto Method # 1: The standard ketogenic diet (SKD) consists of high-fat, moderate protein, and is low in carbs.

Keto Method # 2: Workout times will call for the targeted keto diet, which is also called TKD. The process consists of adding additional carbohydrates to the diet plan during the times when you are more active.

Keto Method # 3: The cyclical ketogenic diet (CKD) entails a restricted five-day keto diet plan, followed by two high-carbohydrate days.

Keto Method 4: The high-protein keto diet is comparable to the standard keto plan (SKD) in all aspects. You will consume more protein.

Macro Guidelines

Ketogenic 0-20 Carbs Daily: Generally, this low level of carbs is related to a restrictive medical diet, where the patient is restricted to <u>10 to 15</u> grams each day to ensure the proper levels of ketosis remains. The Charlie Foundation is one of the plans used to promote the treatment of epilepsy.

Moderate 20-50 Daily Carbs Allowed: If you have diabetes, are obese, or metabolically deranged, this is the plan for you. If you are consuming less than 50 grams daily, your body will achieve a ketosis state, which supplies the ketone bodies.

Liberal 50-100 Daily Carbs Allowed: This option is best if you're active and lean and are attempting to maintain your weight.

Calorie Counting Versus Micros

The short of counting calories is that they don't tell the whole story. You can fill up on the "right" calories, and you may also lose muscle mass. For example, you count one hundred calories of avocado (a fat), which is better than one hundred calories from a cookie (carbs). That is why keto counts the macros (fat, protein, and carbs), not the calories.

Remember This Formula: You will need to calculate your net carbs on some of the recipes you discover on the Internet; some list only the total carbs. If that happens, just take the total carbs listed (-) fiber (=) the total net carb, which is what you need to track an accurate count, so you can remain in ketosis.

Foods Included in the Intermittent Fasting Plan

Fresh Vegetables

You need to add plenty of veggies to your lunch or dinner menu plans. Each of these has the Net Carbs listed per 100 grams or 1/2 cup serving:

- Alfalfa Seeds – Sprouted – 0.2
- Arugula – 2.05
- Asparagus - 6 spears – 2.4
- Hass Avocado – ½ of 1 – 1.8
- Bamboo shoots – 3
- Beans – Green snap – 3.6

- Beet greens – 0.63
- Bell pepper – 2.1
- Broccoli – 4.04
- Cabbage – Savoy – 3
- Carrots – 6.78
- Carrots – baby – 5.34
- Cauliflower – 2.97
- Celery – 1.37
- Chard – 2.14
- Chicory greens – 0.7
- Chives – 1.85
- Coriander – Cilantro leaves – 0.87
- Cucumber with peel – 3.13
- Eggplant – 2.88
- Garlic – 30.96
- Ginger root – 15.77
- Kale – 5.15
- Leeks – bulb (+) lower leaf – 12.35
- Lemongrass – citronella – 25.3
- Lettuce – red leaf – 1.36
- Lettuce – e.g., iceberg – 1.77
- Mushrooms brown – 3.7
- Mustard greens – 1.47
- Onions – yellow – 7.64
- Onions – scallions or spring – 4.74
- Onions – sweet – 6.65
- Peppers – banana – 1.95
- Peppers – red hot chili – 7.31
- Peppers – jalapeno – 3.7
- Peppers – sweet – green – 2.94

- Peppers – sweet – red – 3.93
- Peppers – sweet – yellow – 5.42
- Portabella mushrooms – 2.57
- Pumpkin – 6
- Radishes – 1.8
- Seaweed – kelp – 8.27
- Seaweed – spirulina - 2.02
- Shiitake mushrooms – 4.29
- Spinach – 1.43
- Squash – crookneck – summer – 2.64
- Squash – winter – acorn – 8.92
- Tomatoes – 2.69
- Turnips – 4.63
- Turnip greens – 3.93
- Summer squash - 2.6
- Raw watercress - 3.57
- White mushrooms – 2.26
- Zucchini – 1.5

Chili Peppers: The chemical found in chili peppers is called capsaicin, which will boost your metabolism. The capsaicin will increase the fat and calories you burn during your intermittent fasting plan.

Twenty research studies indicated that you would lose/burn approximately fifty extra calories daily. However, all researchers now agree with the theory. At any rate, enjoy the chili peppers.

Fresh Fruits

It is essential to eat plenty of fruits while on the ketogenic diet plan.

Enjoy these according to your daily limits of carbohydrates. This collection of keto fruits are 100 grams each for each 1/2 cup serving:

- Apples – no skin, boiled – 13.6 total carbs
- Apricots – 7.5 total carbs
- Bananas – 23.4 total carbs
- Fresh Blackberries – 5.4 net carbs
- Fresh Blueberries – 8.2 net carbs
- Fresh Strawberries – 3 net carbs
- Cantaloupe – 6 total carbs
- Raw Cranberries – 4 net carbs
- Gooseberries – 8.8 net carbs
- Kiwi – 14.2 total carbs
- Fresh Boysenberries – 8.8 net carbs
- Oranges – 11.7 total carbs
- Peaches – 11.6 total carbs
- Pears – 19.2 total carbs
- Pineapple – 11 total carbs
- Plums – 16.3 total carbs
- Watermelon – 7.1 total carbs

Excellent Spices

Black Pepper: Pepper promotes nutrient absorption in the tissues all over your body, speeds up your metabolism, and improves digestion. The main ingredient of pepper is alkaloid piperine, which gives it the pungent taste. It can boost fat metabolism by as much as 8% for up to several hours after it has been ingested.

Basil: (1 whole leaf, 0.5 gram is 0 net carbs) You can use fresh or dried basil to maximize its benefits. Its dark green color is an indication that it also maintains an outstanding source of magnesium, calcium, and vitamin K, which are excellent for your bones. It also helps with allergies, arthritis, or inflammatory bowel
conditions.

Cinnamon: (1 tsp. is 0.6 grams net carbs) Use cinnamon as part of your daily plan to improve your insulin receptor activity. Just put one-half of a teaspoon of cinnamon into a smoothie, shake, or any other dessert.

Raw Ginger Root is *0.9 net carbs for 1 tbsp and involves* over 25 antioxidants. It maintains hefty anti-inflammatory elements to help reduce muscle aches and the pain and swelling of arthritis. Ginger is best known for its ability to reduce nausea and vomiting and its soothing remedy for sore throats from outbreaks of flu and colds. Have a tea made with hot water simmered with a small amount of lemon and honey and a few slices of ginger as a soothing tonic when you're sick.

Cumin Powder: (1 tbsp. is <u>2 grams net carbs</u>) Cumin maintains abundant antioxidants which are excellent for your <u>digestion</u> and so much more. It also stimulates the pancreas and gallbladder to secrete bile and enzymes which work to break down the food into usable nutrients your body needs to function healthily. Cumin also helps detoxify the body and is beneficial for several respiratory disorders, including bronchitis and asthma. Cumin is also an excellent source of vitamin A & C, as well as iron, which are all excellent for your immune system.

Cloves: Cloves possess a spicy and sweet flavor, but they also contain powerful natural medicine, including strong antiseptic and germicidal components that can help ward off arthritis pain, gum and tooth pain, and infections. They also relieve digestive problems.

Acceptable Sweeteners

Swerve Granular Sweetener is an excellent choice as a blend. It's made from non-digestible carbs sourced from starchy root veggies and select fruits. Start with 3/4 of a teaspoon for every one teaspoon of sugar. Increase the portion to your taste.

Stevia Drops offer delicious flavors, including hazelnut, vanilla, English toffee, and chocolate. Some individuals think the drops are too bitter, so use only three drops at first to equal one teaspoon of sugar.

Xylitol is at the top of the sugar alternatives, which is an excellent choice to sweeten your teriyaki and barbecue sauce. Its naturally occurring sugar alcohol has a glycemic index (GI) standing of 13.

Beverage Options

Coffee: Your caffeine levels can help increase the metabolic rate by approximately 11%. Studies have shown consumption of a minimum of 270 mg of caffeine—about three cups of coffee—will burn away an additional 100 calories daily. The rates can surely boost your intermittent fasting, as long as you leave it sugar-free.

Tea: Tea is offered as a good source of beverage because of the catechins in the tea conglomerate with the caffeine to help speed up your metabolism. The catechins are an antioxidant and a type of natural phenol which is from the chemical family of flavonoids.

An additional 100 calories can be burned daily to increase your metabolism by four to ten percent with the use of green and oolong tea. The effects may be different with each fasting participant.

Include Healthy Fats & Oils

Extra-Virgin Olive Oil (EVOO): Olive oil dates back to centuries, back when oil was used for anointing kings and priests.

High-quality oil with its low acidity makes the oil have a smoke point as high as 410° Fahrenheit. That's higher than most cooking applications call for, making olive oil more heat-stable than many other cooking fats. It contains (2 tsp.) -0- carbs.

Monounsaturated fats, such as the ones in olive oil, are also linked with better blood sugar regulation, including lower fasting glucose, as well as reducing inflammation throughout the body.

Olive oil also helps prevent cardiovascular disease by protecting the integrity of your vascular system and lowering LDL, which is also called the "bad" cholesterol.

Coconut Oil: You vamp up the fat intake with this high flash-point oil. Enjoy a coconut oil smoothie before your workouts.

Use it with your meats, chicken, fish, or on top of veggies. It will quickly transfer from solid form to oil according to its temperature.

Other Monounsaturated & Saturated Fats

Include these items (listed in grams):

- Avocado, Sesame, Olive, & Flaxseed Oil – 1 tbsp. – 0–net carbs
- Olives – 3 jumbo – 5 large or 10 small – 1 net carb
- Chicken fat, Beef tallow & Duck fat – 1 tbsp. – 0 net carbs
- Unsweetened flaked coconut – 3 tbsp. – 2 net carbs
- Ghee & Unsalted Butter – 1 tbsp. – 0 net carbs
- Egg yolks – 1 large – 0.6 net carbs
- Organic Red Palm oil – e.g., Nutiva - 1 tbsp. – 0 – net carbs

- Various Dressings
- Keto-Friendly Mayonnaise

Other Choices for the Ketogenic Plan

- *Grass-Fed Butter:* You can promote fat loss with butter that is almost carb-free. The butter is a naturally occurring fatty acid which is rich in conjugated linoleic acid (CLA). It is suitable for maintaining weight loss and retaining lean muscle mass.
- *Ghee* is also a great staple for your keto stock, which is also called clarified butter.
- *Yogurt:* Coconut milk is easily digested and contains fats, including lauric acid. Yogurt provides transient bacteria since it feeds existing healthy gut bacteria as they pass through your intestinal tract.

Include These Cold Items

- Full-fat sour cream
- Goat cheese
- Full-fat cream cheese
- Parmesan cheese
- Hard & soft cheeses, e.g., mozzarella or sharp cheddar

CHAPTER 2:

How to Get Started on the 16/8 Plan

You will still be able to enjoy your regular meals, except you are eating in the eight-hour window.

How to Begin

Step 1: Choose a non-stressful week to begin the ketogenic diet plan.

Step 2: Purge the pantry and fridge.

Step 3: Restock the fridge and pantry with ketogenic food items.

Step 4: Consider skipping one meal each day. Maybe sleep a little longer and have brunch.

Step 5: Initially, don't exceed your net carbs and don't limit the fat and protein you consume.

Step 6: Make a routine. Drink a large glass of water and have a supplement of a ½ teaspoon of MCT oil or 2 teaspoons of coconut oil.

Step 7: Keep track of your ketone levels.

Once you have set your goals and calculated how many carbs you are allowed in one day, it is time to explore the Lean-Gains Method fully. The 16/8 Method is also called the Lean-Gains Method. The plan is used as a routine targeted explicitly for the removal of body fat and to improve lean muscle mass. One of the most noteworthy benefits of this type of fasting is that it's incredibly flexible so that it will work well if you have a varied schedule. This safe program provides a fasting window of 16 hours, with hours of eating at 8 hours. The easiest way to attempt this schedule is to stop eating after dinner in the evening and wait 14 hours, which means skipping breakfast and picking things up in the early afternoon. For women, you'll fast for 14 hours compared to 16 hours for men before allowing a reasonable quantity of calories for the remaining 8 to 10 hours. Most people find it helpful to either eat two large meals during the 8 or 10-hour feeding period or split that time into three smaller meals since that is the way most people are already programmed.

A study was performed by the Obesity Society, stating that if you have your dinner before 2:00 p.m., your hunger yearnings will be reduced for the remainder of the day. At the same time, your fat-burning reserves are boosted. During the fasting period, you should only consume food items that have zero calories, including black coffee (a splash of cream is excellent), water, diet soda, and sugar-free gum.

Avoid These Food Items

- *Processed Meats:* While protein is an undeniably important part of a healthy diet, seeking your protein from meats, which have been treated, will overload your body full of chemicals. The processed meats tend to be lower in protein while higher in sodium and contain preservatives that can cause a variety of health risks, including asthma and heart disease. Choose from the quality cuts of meat found in most grocery stores.

- *White Flour:* Much like processed meats, by the time white flour has completed the processing, it's utterly devoid of any nutritional value. According to *Care2*, white flour, when consumed as part of a regular diet, has been shown to increase a woman's chance of breast cancer by a shocking 200%.

- *Non-Organic Milk:* Despite being touted as part of a balanced diet, non-organic milk is routinely found to be full of growth hormones. The growth hormones leave behind antibiotics, which, in turn, makes it more difficult for the human body to counter infections, causing an increased chance of colon cancer, prostate cancer, and breast cancer.

- *Farm-Raised Salmon:* Much like processed meat, farm-raised salmons are the least healthy type of an otherwise healthy meal choice. When salmons are raised in close proximity to one another for a prolonged period, they lose much of their natural vitamin D while picking up traces of PCB, DDT, carcinogens, and bromine.

- *Non-Organic Potatoes:* While the starch and carbohydrates it contains are a vital part of a balanced meal, non-organic potatoes are not worth the trouble. They are treated with chemicals while still in the ground, before being treated again; they are sent to the store as "fresh" as possible. These chemicals have been shown to increase the risk of things like birth defects, autism, asthma, learning disabilities, Parkinson's, and

Alzheimer's disease, as well as multiple types of cancer.

Now that you have a good idea of how to proceed with your new way of eating, it is time to review all of the recipes.

CHAPTER 3:

Breakfast Favorites

1. *Almond Coconut Egg Wraps*

Serving Yields Provided: 4

Macro Counts - Each Serving:

- Net Carbs: 3 g
- Total Fats: 8 g
- Protein: 8 g
- Calories: 111

Ingredients Needed:

- Organic eggs (5)
- Almond meal (2 tbsp.)
- Sea salt (.25 tsp.)
- Coconut flour (1 tbsp.)

Directions for Preparation:

1. Combine the fixings in a blender and work until creamy.
2. Warm up a skillet using the medium-high temperature setting.

3. Pour 2 tbsp of batter into the pan and cover with a top.

4. Simmer for about 3 minutes.

5. Flip it over and continue cooking for an additional 3 minutes.

6. Serve hot.

2. *Almonds & Chips Breakfast Cereal*

Serving Yields Provided: 1

Macro Counts - Each Serving:

- Net Carbs: 3 g
- Protein: 6 g
- Total Fats: 27 g
- Calories: 300

Ingredients Needed:

- Coconut milk (.25 cup)
- Hemp hearts (3 tbsp.)
- Shredded coconut (.5 tbsp.)
- Chocolate chips (.5 tbsp.)
- Chopped almonds (.5 tbsp.)
- Liquid stevia (1 drop)

Directions for Preparation:

1. Store in the refrigerator for at least 4 hrs. Overnight is best.
2. Enjoy cold or warm.

3. *Almost McGriddle Casserole*

Serving Yields Provided: 8

Macro Counts - Each Serving:

- Net Carbs: 3 g
- Total Fats: 36 g
- Protein: 26 g
- Calories: 448

Ingredients Needed:

- Breakfast sausage (1 lb.)
- Flaxseed meal (.25 cup)
- Almond flour (1 cup)
- Large eggs (10)
- Maple syrup (6 tbsp.)
- Cheese (4 oz.)
- Butter (4 tbsp.)
- Onion (.5 tsp.)
- Sage (.25 tsp.)
- Garlic powder (.5 tsp.)
- *Also Needed*: 9 x 9-inch casserole dish & parchment baking paper

Directions for Preparation:

1. Heat the oven temperature to 350° Fahrenheit.

2. Use the medium heat setting on the stovetop to prepare the sausage in a skillet.

3. Add all of the dry ingredients (the cheese also), and stir in the wet ones. Add 4 tablespoons of the syrup. Stir and blend well.

4. After the sausage has browned, combine all of the fixings, along with the grease.

5. Prepare the casserole dish with a layer of baking paper. Empty the mix into the casserole dish and drizzle the rest of the syrup.

6. Bake for 45–55 minutes.

7. Transfer to the countertop and let it become room temperature. The casserole should be easy to remove by using the edge of the parchment paper.

4. *Bacon Hash*

Serving Yields Provided: 2

Macro Counts - Each Serving:

- Net Carbs: 9 g
- Total Fats: 24 g
- Protein: 23 g
- Calories: 366

Ingredients Needed:

- Bacon slices (6)
- Small onion (1)
- Small green pepper (1)
- Jalapenos (2)
- Eggs (4)

Directions for Preparation:

1. Chop the bacon into chunks using a food processor. Set aside for now.
2. Slice the peppers and onions into thin strips, and dice the jalapenos as small as possible.
3. Prepare a skillet with a spritz of non-stick cooking oil spray and fry the veggies.

4. Once browned, combine all of the fixings and cook until crispy.
5. Place on a serving dish with the eggs.

5. *Bagels & Cheese*

Serving Yields Provided: 6

Macro Counts - Each Serving:

- Net Carbs: 8 g
- Total Fats: 31 g
- Protein: 19 g
- Calories: 374

Ingredients Needed:

- Cream cheese (3 oz.)
- Baking powder (1 tsp.)
- Shredded mozzarella cheese (2.5 cups)
- Almond flour (1.5 cups)
- Eggs (2)

Directions for Preparation:

1. Combine the baking powder, mozzarella, flour, and cream cheese in a mixing container. Place in the microwave to melt for about 1 minute. Stir well.
2. Let the mixture cool and add the eggs. Break apart into six sections and shape into round bagels.
3. *Note*: You can also sprinkle with a seasoning of your choice or pinch of salt if desired.

4. Bake until the edges of the bagels are golden brown (12 to 15 min.).
5. Cool and store.

6. _Belgian Style Waffles_

Serving Yields Provided: 4

Macro Counts - Each Serving:
- Net Carbs: 3 g
- Total Fats: 19g
- Protein: 11 g
- Calories: 247

Ingredients Needed:
- Melted butter or ghee (4 tbsp.)
- Eggs (6)
- Salt (.5 tsp.)
- Bak. powder (.5 tsp.)
- Coconut flour (.33 cup)
- _Optional:_ Sweet Leaf stevia drops (.125 tsp.)

Directions for Preparation:
1. In a blender, mix the butter and eggs until incorporated.
2. Pour in the salt, stevia, and baking powder. Blend well to combine.
3. Fold in the flour, and let it rest to thicken (5 min.)
4. Pour in small amounts of water as needed to thin the batter.
5. Prepare in the waffle maker and serve.

7. *Biscuits & Gravy*

Serving Yields Provided: 2

Macro Counts - Each Serving:

- Net Carbs: 2 g
- Total Fats: 36 g
- Protein: 22 g
- Calories: 425

Ingredients Needed:

- Salt (.25 tsp.)
- Almond flour (.25 cup)
- Baking powder (.5 tsp.)
- Large egg white (1)
- Crumbled breakfast sausage (6 oz.)
- Chicken broth (.25 cup)
- Cream cheese (.25 cup)
- Pepper & Salt (to your liking)

Directions for Preparation:

1. Warm up the oven to 400° Fahrenheit.
2. Prepare a baking tin with parchment baking paper.
3. Whisk the salt, almond flour, and baking powder.
4. In another dish, whisk the egg whites to form stiff peaks.

5. Dice the butter into small bits. Form a crumbled mixture in the dry components using the butter. Gently blend it into the egg whites.

6. Split the mixture of batter into two portions on the paper-lined pan. Bake for 11 to 15 minutes.

7. Using the medium heat setting, warm the sausage. When browned, add the cream cheese and chicken broth. Simmer and dust with pepper and salt.

8. Serve with the piping hot biscuits with a serving of the delicious gravy.

8. _Blueberry Flaxseed Muffins_

Serving Yields Provided: 10

Macro Counts - Each Serving:

- Net Carbs: 8.78 g
- Total Fats: 18.3g
- Protein: 7.57 g
- Calories: 221

Ingredients Needed:

- Flaxseeds (1.5 cups)
- Baking powder (1 tbsp.)
- Eggs (5)
- Vanilla extract (1 tsp.)
- Almond milk (3 tbsp.)
- Coconut oil (4 tbsp.)
- Blueberries (.5 cup)
- Salt (1 pinch)
- Sugar substitute (to your liking)

Directions for Preparation:

1. Warm up the oven to reach 350° Fahrenheit.
2. Use a coffee grinder to prepare the seeds.
3. Combine each of the dry fixings in a mixing container.

4. Whisk the eggs in a mixing container. Pour in the oil and milk. Stir well.
5. Combine all of the fixings.
6. Fold in the berries and stir gently with a spoon.
7. Pour into muffin cups.
8. Bake for 15 minutes. Cool slightly and serve.

9. *Blueberry Ricotta Pancakes*

Serving Yields Provided: 5

Macro Counts - Each Serving:

- Net Carbs: 6 g
- Total Fats: 23 g
- Protein: 15 g
- Calories: 311

Ingredients Needed:

- Ricotta (.75 cup)
- Large eggs (3)
- Unsweetened vanilla almond milk (.25 cup)
- Golden flaxseed meal (.5 cup)
- Salt (.25 tsp.)
- Baking powder (1 tsp.)
- Almond flour (1 cup)
- Stevia powder (.5 tsp.)
- Vanilla extract (.5 tsp.)
- Blueberries (.25 cup)
- *Optional*: Keto-friendly syrup of choice; add the carbs

Directions for Preparation:

1. Blend the eggs, milk, ricotta, and vanilla extract with an electric mixer.

2. Combine the flaxseed meal, salt, flour, baking powder, and stevia in another dish.

3. Add the dry ingredients into the blender—slowly—to form the batter. Use two to three blueberries for each pancake.

4. Add the butter to a preheated skillet using a medium heat setting. When it melts, add the batter using two tablespoons for each scoop.

5. At this point, serve or set aside to cool.

6. You can serve or freeze to use later if you have limited time. If you know your schedule will be rushed, you can pour the syrup in a cup with a lid.

7. Enjoy with a side of bacon, but add the additional carbs to the count.

10.   *Chocolate Loaf*

Serving Yields Provided: 8

Macro Counts - Each Serving:

- Net Carbs: 2.32 g
- Total Fats: 17.8g
- Protein: 5.7 g
- Calories: 195

Ingredients Needed:

- Large eggs (6)
- Coconut flour (.75 cup)
- Butter (4 oz.)
- Unsweetened cocoa powder (.33 cup)
- Bak. soda (.5 tsp.)
- Salt (1 pinch)
- Bak. powder (1 tsp.)
- Sugar substitute (as desired)
- Apple cider vinegar (2 tsp.)
- *Also Needed*: Parchment paper

Directions for Preparation:

1. Warm the oven to reach 350° Fahrenheit.
2. Line the baking pan with the paper.
3. Whisk the eggs and stir in the melted butter.

4. Sift the dry fixings. Pour in the wet mixture, and add the vinegar.

5. Stir well and pour into the pan.

6. Bake for 20 to 30 minutes.

7. Serve after testing its doneness (if the toothpick inserted in the center comes out clean.

11.   *Cinnamon Raisin Bagels*

Serving Yields Provided: 6

Macro Counts - Each Serving:

- Net Carbs: 6 g
- Total Fats: 10 g
- Protein: 3 g
- Calories: 139

Ingredients Needed:

- Coconut flour sifted (.33 cup)
- Golden flax meal (1.5 tbsp.)
- Baking soda (.5 tsp.)
- *Optional:* Sea salt (a dash)
- Baking powder (1 tsp.)
- Cinnamon (2 tsp.)
- Whisked eggs (3)
- Apple cider vinegar (1 tsp.)
- Unsweetened coconut or almond milk (.33 cup)
- Melted butter - coconut oil or ghee (2.5 tbsp.)
- Liquid stevia (1 tsp.)
- Golden raisins (.33 cup)
- *Optional*: Vanilla extract (1 tsp.)
- *Also Needed:* Donut/bagel pan

Directions for Preparation:

1. Warm up the oven to 350° Fahrenheit.

2. Grease the pan.

3. Mix the dry fixings (the golden flax meal, the sifted coconut flour, baking soda, cinnamon, sea salt, and baking powder) thoroughly.

4. In another container, combine the almond/coconut milk, apple cider vinegar, eggs, melted butter/coconut oil, vanilla extract, and stevia.

5. Combine all of the fixings and add to the prepared pan, spreading evenly with a spatula.

6. Bake for 17 to 20 minutes. Cool for 3 to 4 minutes.

7. Loosen the bagels with a knife. Turn the bread on the side and slice into half.

8. Serve with toppings of your choice, such as butter or cream cheese.

9. Refrigerate or freeze unused portions.

12.   *<u>Classic Bacon & Eggs</u>*

Serving Yields Provided:

Macro Counts - Each Serving:

- Net Carbs: 1 g
- Total Fats: 22 g
- Protein: 15g
- Calories: 272

Ingredients Needed:

- Eggs (8)
- Sliced bacon (5 oz.)
- *Optional:* Cherry tomatoes & Fresh parsley

Directions for Preparation:

1. Prepare the bacon in a skillet using the medium-high temperature until crispy. Leave the rendered fat in the pan, and put the bacon in a platter to drain.
2. Fry the eggs in the bacon remnants using medium heat.
3. Cook the eggs any way you like them. For a *Sunny Side Up*, leave the eggs to fry on one side. Cover the pan with a lid to make sure they get cooked on top. For *Over-Easy Eggs*, flip the eggs over after a few minutes and cook for another minute.

4. Slice the cherry tomatoes in half, and fry them at the same time.

5. Dust with pepper and salt to your liking.

13.   *Cocoa Waffles*

Serving Yields Provided: 5

Macro Counts - Each Serving:

- Net Carbs: 3.4 g
- Protein: 7 g
- Total Fats: 27 g
- Calories: 289

Ingredients Needed:

- Separated eggs (5)
- Unsweetened cocoa (.25 cup)
- Granular sweetener (3 tbsp.)
- Coconut flour (4 tbsp.)
- Baking powder (1 tsp.)
- Melted butter (4.5 oz.)
- Milk of choice (3 tbsp.)
- Vanilla (1 tsp.)

Directions for Preparation:

1. Use a whisk to prepare the egg whites. Briskly mix to form stiff peaks.
2. In another container, whisk the sweetener, baking powder, and cocoa with the egg yolks.

3. Add the butter to the dry mixture. Stir in the vanilla and milk.
4. Fold in the prepared egg whites, a little at a time.
5. Transfer the mixture in the waffle maker.
6. Cook until they are golden brown.
7. Serve.

CHAPTER 4:

Lunchtime Options

14.   *Bread Twists for the Salad*

Serving Yields Provided: 10

Macro Counts - Each Serving:

- Net Carbs: 1 g
- Total Fats: 18 g
- Protein: 7 g
- Calories: 204

Ingredients Needed:

- Almond flour (.5 cup)
- Coconut flour (4 tbsp.)
- Salt (.5 tsp.)
- Baking powder (1 tsp.)
- Shredded cheese, your choice (1.5 cups)
- Butter (2.33 oz.)
- Egg (2, use 1 for brushing the tops)
- Green pesto (2 oz.)

Directions for Preparation:

1. Warm up the oven to reach 350° Fahrenheit. Prepare a cookie sheet with a layer of parchment paper.
2. Mix all of the dry fixings.
3. Use the low heat setting to melt the butter and cheese together. Stir until smooth and add the egg. Stir well.
4. Combine all of the fixings to make the dough.
5. Roll out the dough between the two layers of parchment paper until it is about 1-inch thick. Remove the top sheet.
6. Spread the pesto on top of the dough and slice into 1-inch strips.
7. Twist the dough and arrange on the baking tin. Brush the twists with the second egg (gently whisked).
8. Bake until golden brown, about 15 to 20 minutes.

15.   *Caprese Salad*

Serving Yields Provided: 4

Macro Counts - Each Serving:

- Net Carbs: 4.6 g
- Total Fats: 63.5 g
- Protein: 7.7 g
- Calories: 191

Ingredients Needed:

- Grape tomatoes (3 cups)
- Peeled garlic cloves (4)
- Avocado oil (2 tbsp.)
- Mozzarella balls (10 pearl-sized)
- Baby spinach leaves (4 cups)
- Fresh basil leaves (.25 cup)
- Brine reserved from the cheese (1 tbsp.)
- Pesto (1 tbsp.)

Directions for Preparation:

1. Program the oven setting to 400° Fahrenheit.
2. Prepare a baking tin with a layer of aluminum foil.

3. Arrange the tomatoes and cloves in the prepared pan. Spritz with the oil. Bake 20-30 minutes or until the tops are slightly browned.
4. Drain the liquid (saving 1 tbsp) from the brine. Mix the pesto with the brine.
5. Arrange the spinach in a large salad container. Transfer the tomatoes to the dish, along with the roasted garlic. Drizzle with the pesto sauce.
6. Garnish with the mozzarella balls and freshly torn basil leaves.

16.   *Chicken BLT Salad*

Serving Yields Provided: 4

Macro Counts - Each Serving:

- Net Carbs: 4 g
- Total Fats: 78g
- Protein: 28 g
- Calories: 837

Ingredients Needed:

- Boneless chicken thighs (1 lb.)
- Butter (1 oz.)
- Bacon (.5 lb.)
- Cherry tomatoes (4 oz.)
- Romaine lettuce (10 oz.)
- Salt and pepper (to your liking)

Ingredients Needed - Garlic Mayonnaise:

- Mayonnaise (.75 cup)
- Garlic powder (.5 tbsp.)

Directions for Preparation:

1. Whisk the mayonnaise and garlic powder in a small bowl and set aside for now.

2. Fry the bacon in butter until crispy. Transfer to a dish to drain and keep warm. Save the grease in the pan.
3. Shred the chicken and dust using the salt and pepper. Fry in the same skillet as the bacon until golden brown.
4. Rinse and shred the lettuce.
5. Toss the lettuce on a plate and top with chicken, bacon, tomatoes, and a serving of garlic mayonnaise.

17. *Chicken, Feta, & Kiwi Salad*

Serving Yields Provided: 2

Macro Counts - Each Serving:
- Net Carbs: 13 g
- Total Fats: 15 g
- Protein: 28 g
- Calories: 314

Ingredients Needed:
- Fig balsamic vinegar (1 tbsp.)
- Kiwis (2)
- Extra-virgin olive oil (1 tbsp.)
- Salt (1 pinch)
- Mixed field greens (4 cups)
- Chopped grilled chicken breast (1 cup, about 5 oz.)
- Feta cheese (.33 cup)

Directions for Preparation:
1. Chop the chicken and crumble the feta.
2. Whisk the balsamic vinegar, oil, and salt.
3. Add the greens and chicken breast.
4. Peel and cut the kiwi into halves. Dice into 1-inch wedges and add to the salad with the crumbled feta.
5. Toss well to combine.

18.   *Chicken-Pecan Salad & Cucumber Bites*

Serving Yields Provided: 2

Macro Counts - Each Serving:

- Net Carbs: 3 g
- Total Fats: 24 g
- Protein: 23 g
- Calories: 323

Ingredients Needed:

- Mayonnaise (2 tbsp.)
- Precooked chicken breast (1 cup)
- Cucumber (1)
- Diced celery (.25 cup)
- Chopped pecans (.25 cup)
- Pink salt—Himalayan & Black pepper (1 pinch of each)

Directions for Preparation:

1. Peel and slice the cucumber into 1/4-inch slices. Dice the chicken and celery. Chop the pecans.
2. Combine the pecans, chicken, mayo, and celery in a salad bowl. Sprinkle with pepper and salt.

3. Lay the cucumber slices on a platter, and add a pinch of salt. Layer each one with a spoonful of the chicken salad. Serve.

19.   *Cobb Salad*

Serving Yields Provided: 2

Macro Counts - Each Serving:

- Net Carbs: 3 g
- Total Fats: 48 g
- Protein: 43 g
- Calories: 600

Ingredients Needed:

- Hard-boiled egg (1)
- Spinach (1 cup)
- Bacon strips (2)
- Campari tomato (.5 of 1)
- Chicken breast (2 oz.)
- Avocado (.25 of 1)
- Olive oil (1 tbsp.)
- White vinegar (.5 tsp.)

Directions for Preparation:

1. Prepare the bacon and chicken shred or slice the chicken.

2. Cut all of the ingredients into small pieces.
3. Toss them to a bowl with the vinegar and oil. Toss gently and serve.

20.   *Egg Salad*

Serving Yields Provided: 4

Macro Counts - Each Serving:

- Net Carbs: 1.4 g
- Total Fats: 29 g
- Protein: 8.7 g
- Calories: 305

Ingredients Needed:

- Hard-boiled eggs (6)
- Curry Powder (1 tsp. or to taste)
- Full-fat Mayonnaise (.5 cup)

Directions for Preparation:

1. Prepare the boiled eggs by adding them into a saucepan. Pour in *cold* water.
2. Turn the burner on.
3. Once the water begins to boil, set a timer for 7 minutes and then pour the hot water when done.
4. Prepare a cold-water bath, and submerge the hot eggs into it to stop the cooking process.

5. When cooled, peel and chop the eggs into small bits.

6. Combine the mayo, eggs, and curry powder.

7. Serve with a portion of chopped fresh parsley.

21. *Greek Salad*

Serving Yields Provided: 1

Macro Counts - Each Serving:
- Net Carbs: 8 g
- Total Fats: 57.5 g
- Protein: 12 g
- Calories: 594

Ingredients Needed:
- Red onion (.25 cup)
- Tomato (.25 cup)
- Olive oil (3 tbsp.)
- Cucumber (.25 cup)
- Bell pepper (.25 cup)
- Feta cheese (.5 cup)
- Olives (1 tbsp.)
- Red wine vinegar (.5 tbsp.)

Directions for Preparation:

1. Dice the tomato, chop the olives, and slice the onion, cucumber, and pepper. Combine the bell pepper with the tomato, cucumber, crumbled feta cheese, and onion.

2. Spritz using the oil and vinegar with a shake of pepper and salt to your liking.

3. Toss until all of the ingredients are mixed well before serving.

Soup Choices

22.   *Broccoli Curry Soup*

Serving Yields Provided: 4

Macro Counts - Each Serving:
- Net Carbs: 4.8 g
- Total Fats: 19.8 g
- Protein: 16.9 g
- Calories: 375

Ingredients Needed:
- Salt & Black pepper (as needed)
- Onion (1)
- Curry (1 tbsp.)
- Coconut oil (2 tbsp.)
- Vegetable stock (1 liter)
- Coconut cream (1 cup)
- Keto-friendly sharp cheese, your choice (.75 cup)
- Broccoli (1 lb.)

Directions for Preparation:

1. Pour the coconut oil into a frying pan on the stovetop over a burner turned to the medium-high heat setting.

2. Chop the onion and add to the pan. Simmer for approximately 6 minutes.

3. Lower the temperature to medium. Then, add in the broth until it begins to simmer. Mix in the broccoli, as well as any seasonings before adding in the curry and letting it simmer for 20 minutes.

4. Pour into a blender before mixing in the cheese substitute.

5. Blend well.

23.   *Chicken Chowder – Crockpot*

Serving Yields Provided: 4

Macro Counts - Each Serving:

- Net Carbs: 7.5 g
- Total Fats: 28.8 g
- Protein: 40 g
- Calories: 457

Ingredients Needed:

- Garlic clove (1)
- Cilantro (1 tbsp.)
- Small onion (1)
- Cream cheese (8 oz.)
- Chicken broth (1 cup)
- Chicken breasts (1 lb.)
- Diced tomatoes (14 oz.)
- Diced jalapeno (.5 oz.)
- Fresh lime juice (1.6 oz.)
- Black pepper (1 tbsp.)
- Salt (1 tsp.)

Directions for Preparation:

1. Remove the skin and bones from the chicken.
2. Chop the garlic and cilantro. Dice the onion and jalapeno.
3. Combine all of the fixings in the crockpot.
4. Prepare using the low-temperature setting for 6 to 9 hours or high for 4 hours.
5. Once it is done, shred the chicken in the pot using two forks.
6. Serve and enjoy.

Seafood

24.   _Alfredo Shrimp_

Serving Yields Provided: 4

Macro Counts - Each Serving:

- Net Carbs: 6.5 g
- Total Fats: 18 g
- Protein: 23 g
- Calories: 298

Ingredients Needed:

- Raw shrimp (1 lb.)
- Salted butter (1 tbsp.)
- Cubed cream cheese (4 oz.)
- Whole milk (.5 cup)
- Dried basil (1 tsp.)
- Salt (1 tsp.)
- Garlic powder (1 tbsp.)
- Shredded parmesan cheese (.5 cup)
- Baby kale or spinach (.25 cup)

- Whole sun-dried tomatoes (5)
- *Also Needed:* Food processor or blender

Directions for Preparation:

1. Heat the butter using the medium heat setting in a skillet.
2. Toss in the shrimp and lower the heat to medium-low.
3. After 30 seconds, flip the shrimp and cook until slightly pink. Blend in the cream cheese.
4. Increase the heat, and pour in the milk. Stir frequently.
5. Sprinkle with the salt, basil, and garlic. Empty the parmesan cheese in and mix well.
6. Simmer until the sauce has thickened. Cut the sun-dried tomatoes into strips.
7. Lastly, fold in the kale/spinach and sun-dried tomatoes. Serve steaming hot.

25.   *Avocado & Salmon Omelet Wrap*

Serving Yields Provided: 2

Macro Counts - Each Serving:

- Net Carbs: 5.8 g
- Total Fats: 66.9 g
- Protein: 36.9 g
- Calories: 765

Ingredients Needed:

- Large eggs (3)
- Smoked salmon (1.8 oz.)
- Avocado (.5 of 1 average-size)
- Spring onion (1)
- Cream cheese - full-fat (2 tbsp.)
- Chives, freshly chopped (2 tbsp.)
- Butter or ghee (1 tbsp.)
- Pepper and salt (as desired)

Directions for Preparation:

1. Add a sprinkle of pepper and salt to the eggs. Use a fork or whisk, mixing them well. Blend in the chives and cream cheese.

2. Prepare the salmon and avocado (peel and slice or chop).

3. Combine the butter/ghee and the egg mixture in a frying pan. Continue cooking on low heat until done.

4. Place the omelet on a serving dish with a portion of cheese over it. Sprinkle the onion, prepared avocado, and salmon into the wrap.

5. Close and serve!

Other Delicious Lunchtime Choices

26. *Buffalo Cauliflower Bites*

Serving Yields Provided: 4

Macro Counts - Each Serving:

- Net Carbs: 3 g
- Total Fats: 12 g
- Protein: 2 g
- Calories: 130

Ingredients Needed:

- Cauliflower florets (4 cups)
- Cracked black pepper (as desired)
- Sea salt (.25 tsp.)
- Cayenne pepper (.25 tsp.)
- Salted butter (4 tbsp.)
- Hot sauce (.25 cup)
- Minced garlic (1 clove)
- Paprika (.25 tsp.)
- *Optional:* Blue cheese dressing

Directions for Preparation:

1. Warm the oven until it reaches 375° Fahrenheit.

2. Arrange the florets on a paper-lined baking tray.

3. Whisk the cayenne, black pepper, salt, paprika, garlic, butter, and hot sauce. Pour into a microwavable-safe dish for 30 seconds or until smooth.

4. Empty the sauce over the florets in the pan and bake for 25 minutes.

5. Serve with a bowl of blue cheese dressing for dipping.

27.   *Chinese Sauce Fried Rice*

Serving Yields Provided:

Macro Counts - Each Serving:

- Net Carbs: 4.3 g
- Protein: 17 g
- Total Fats: 20.5 g
- Calories: 289

Ingredients Needed:

- Cauliflower (1 medium head)
- Butter (.5 of 1 stick, 4 tbsp.)
- Green onions (2 large)
- Garlic (4 cloves)
- Carrot (.5 cup)
- Yellow & red bell pepper (.5 cup of each)
- Coconut aminos (4 tbsp.)
- Sesame oil (1 tbsp.)
- Sea salt (1 tsp. or more to your liking)
- Crushed red pepper flakes (.5 tsp.)
- Chinese sausage (.5 lb.)
- Frozen peas (.5 cup)
- Large eggs (3)
- *Also Needed*: Box grater or food processor & Wok

Directions for Preparation:

1. Separately chop the white and green parts of the onions. Mince the garlic cloves and dice the peppers. Thinly slice the carrots and sausage.

2. Rice the cauliflower.

3. Warm up the wok using the medium heat setting. In the wok, warm up 1 tablespoon of butter, garlic, and white portion of the onions. Sauté for 2 to 3 minutes.

4. Toss in the rest of the butter, carrot, and bell peppers. Sauté for 5 to 7 minutes.

5. Toss in the sea salt, red pepper flakes, riced cauliflower, coconut aminos, and sesame oil.

6. Stir-fry for about 10 minutes and add the sausage and peas. Stir-fry for another 5 minutes.

7. Push all the fixings in the wok over to one side.

8. Whisk the eggs using a fork and add to the empty side and lightly scramble. Slowly mix them in with the rest of the fixings.

9. Garnish with green onions and serve.

CHAPTER 5:

Tasty Dinner Choices

Poultry

28. *Buffalo Chicken Burgers*

Serving Yields Provided: 2 burgers

Macro Counts - Each Serving:

- Net Carbs: 1 g
- Total Fats: 34 g
- Protein: 43 g
- Calories: 488

Ingredients Needed:

- Cooked chicken breasts (8 oz.)
- Room-temperature cream cheese (2 oz.)
- Shredded mozzarella cheese (.5 cup)
- Frank's Red-Hot Sauce or your choice (2 tbsp.)
- *For Frying*: Ghee or Coconut oil

Directions for Preparation:

1. Either chop or shred the prepared chicken and combine with the rest of the fixings.

2. Place the fixings in the microwave for 15 to 20 seconds to help compact the ingredients. Form two medium patties and place on a plate. Store in the freezer for about 15 minutes.

3. Warm a skillet using the high heat setting. Add the fat and patties. Cook the burgers for 2 to 3 minutes per side.

4. Serve when crispy brown.

29.   *Chicken & Asparagus*

Serving Yields Provided: 8

Macro Counts - Each Serving:

- Net Carbs: 4 g
- Total Fats: 18.2 g
- Protein: 63 g
- Calories: 439

Ingredients Needed:

- Chicken breasts (4 lb.)
- Avocado oil (1 tbsp.)
- Trimmed asparagus (1 lb.)
- Sun-dried tomatoes (4)
- Thick-cut bacon (4 slices)
- Salt (1 tsp.)
- Pepper (.25 tsp.)
- Provolone cheese (8 slices)
- *Also Needed*: 1 baking pan

Directions for Preparation:

1. Set the oven temperature to 400° Fahrenheit.
2. Cut the chicken breasts into eight thin pieces. Chop the bacon and tomatoes into one-inch pieces.

3. Add the oil to the baking pan, along with the chicken and asparagus. Top it off with the tomatoes and bacon.

4. Sprinkle some pepper and salt for seasoning.

5. Bake until the chicken reaches 160º Fahrenheit (internally) or about 25 minutes.

6. Toss in the asparagus and cheese.

7. Garnish with a portion of bacon and tomatoes.

8. Bake for another 3 to 4 minutes until the cheese has melted.

Pork

30. *__BBQ Pork Loin__*

Serving Yields Provided: 4

Macro Counts - Each Serving:

- Net Carbs: 3 g
- Total Fats: 8 g
- Protein: 35 g
- Calories: 238

Ingredients Needed:

- Pork loin (1 lb.)
- Tomato paste (4 tbsp.)
- Worcestershire sauce (1 tsp.)
- Avocado oil (2 tbsp.)
- Smoked paprika (.5 tsp.)
- Minced garlic (.5 tsp.)
- Chopped onion (1 tbsp.)

Directions for Preparation:

1. Whisk the minced garlic, chopped onion, paprika, tomato paste, and Worcestershire sauce.
2. Use the rub to prepare the pork and wrap in foil.
3. Marinate the pork loin in the fridge for at least 1/2 hour for the spices to be absorbed.
4. Add the trivet to the Kitchen robot, and pour the water into the cooker. Secure the lid.
5. Set the timer to 60 minutes. Release the pressure naturally when it's done.
6. Serve.

31. _Carnitas – Crockpot_

Serving Yields Provided: 2

Macro Counts - Each Serving:

- Net Carbs: 4 g
- Total Fats: 26 g
- Protein: 45 g
- Calories: 446

Ingredients Needed:

- Boneless pork butt roast (1 lb.)
- Chili powder (.5 tbsp.)
- Olive oil (1 tbsp.)
- Small diced onion (.5 of 1)
- Minced cloves of garlic (2)
- Juiced lime (1 whole lime)
- Black pepper and Pink salt (as desired)

Directions for Preparation:

1. Use the low-temperature setting to warm up the crockpot.
2. Whisk the olive oil with the chili powder. Rub over the pork and place in the cooker, the fatty side facing up.

3. Prepare the veggies and add along with the lime juice, salt, and pepper.

4. Place the lid on the pot and simmer on low for 8 hours.

5. When ready, shred the meat on a cutting board using two forks.

6. Enjoy on a leaf of lettuce, but remember to add any additional carbs to the carb count.

7. Total prep is just 10 minutes with a cooking time of 8 hrs.

32.   *Crack Slaw – Pork Egg Roll in a Bowl*

Serving Yields Provided: 4

Macro Counts - Each Serving:

- Net Carbs: 5.5 g
- Protein: 20 g
- Total Fats: 20 g
- Calories: 297

Ingredients Needed:

- Sesame oil (2 tbsp.)
- Garlic (3 cloves)
- Yellow onion (.5 cup)
- Green onions, white and green parts (5)
- Ground pork (1 lb.)
- Ground ginger (.5 tsp.)
- Sea salt & black pepper (as desired)
- Sriracha or garlic chili sauce (1 tbsp.)
- Rice vinegar (1 tbsp.)
- Coleslaw mix (14 oz. bag)
- Coconut Aminos (3 tbsp.)
- Toasted sesame seeds (2 tbsp.)

Directions for Preparation:

1. Mince the garlic, and dice the yellow onion. Slice the green onions on the bias.

2. Warm up the oil in a skillet using the medium-high temperature setting.

3. Toss the garlic, white portion of the green onions, and the yellow onions into the pan. Sauté until the onions are translucent and the garlic is fragrant.

4. Add the ground pork, sea salt, black pepper, ground ginger, and Sriracha. Sauté until the pork is fully cooked.

5. Add the coconut aminos, coleslaw mix, and vinegar. Sauté until the coleslaw is tender.

6. Garnish with green onions and sesame seeds before serving.

Fish Seafood Options

33. _Baked Tilapia With Cherry Tomatoes_

Serving Yields Provided: 2
Macro Counts - Each Serving:

- Net Carbs: 4 g

- Total Fats: 8 g

- Protein: 23 g

- Calories: 180

Ingredients Needed:

- Lemon juice (1 tbsp.)

- Butter (2 tsp.)

- Tilapia fillets (2, 4 oz. each)

- Cherry tomatoes (8)

- Pitted black olives (.25 cup)

- Black pepper (.25 tsp.)

- Paprika (.25 tsp.)

- Garlic powder (1 tsp.)

- Salt (.5 tsp.)

- _Optional_: Balsamic vinegar (1 tbsp.)

Directions for Preparation:

1. Set the oven to 375° Fahrenheit.

2. Lightly spritz a roasting pan with some cooking oil. Add the butter, along with the olives and tomatoes in the bottom.

3. Season the tilapia with the spices (paprika, salt, pepper, and garlic powder).

4. Lastly, add the fish fillets with the freshly squeezed lemon juice.

5. Cover the pan with foil and bake until the fish easily flakes (25 to 30 minutes).

6. Garnish with the vinegar if desired.

34.   *Chili Lime Cod*

Serving Yields Provided: 2

Macro Counts - Each Serving:

- Net Carbs: 3 g
- Total Fats: 5 g
- Protein: 37 g
- Calories: 215

Ingredients Needed:

- Wild-caught cod (10–12 oz.)
- Coconut flour (.33 cup)
- Egg (3)
- Lime (1)
- Garlic powder (1 tsp.)
- Cayenne pepper (.5 tsp.)
- Salt (1 tsp.)
- Crushed red pepper (1 tsp.)

Directions for Preparation:

1. Heat the oven temperature to reach 400° Fahrenheit.
2. In separate dishes, whip the egg and remove any lumps from the flour.

3. Let the fillet soak in the egg dish for 1 minute on each side. Add it to the flour dish, and then add it to a baking sheet.

4. Sprinkle the spices and drizzle the lime juice over the cod.

5. Bake it for 10 to 12 minutes or when it easily flakes apart.

6. Drizzle with some Sriracha if you wish, and enjoy.

Beef Options

35. _Bacon Cheeseburger_

Serving Yields Provided: 12

Macro Counts - Each Serving:

- Net Carbs: 0.8 g
- Protein: 27 g
- Total Fats: 41 g
- Calories: 489

Ingredients Needed:

- Low-sodium bacon (16 oz. pkg.)
- Ground beef (3 lb.)
- Eggs (2)
- Medium chopped onion (.5 of 1)
- Shredded cheddar cheese (8 oz.)

Directions for Preparation:

1. Fry the bacon, and chop it into bits. Shred the cheese, and dice the onion.
2. Combine the mixture with the beef and blend in the whisked eggs.

3. Prepare 24 burgers, and grill them the way you like them.

4. You can make a double-decker since they are small. If you like a larger burger, you can just make 12 burgers as a single-decker.

36. *Barbacoa Beef – Kitchen robot*

Serving Yields Provided: 9

Macro Counts - Each Serving:

- Net Carbs: 2 g
- Total Fats: 4.5 g
- Protein: 24 g
- Calories: 153

Ingredients Needed:

- Eye round/bottom round roast (3 lb.)
- Black pepper (as desired)
- Kosher salt (2.5 tsp.)
- Water (1 cup)
- Medium onion (0.5 of 1)
- Lime (1 juiced)
- Garlic cloves (5)
- Chipotles in adobo sauce (2–4)
- Oregano (1 tbsp.)
- Ground cumin (1 tbsp.)
- Oil (1 tsp.)
- Bay leaves (3)
- Ground cloves (0.5 tsp.)

Directions for Preparation:

1. Program the Kitchen robot using the sauté function.

2. Cut the fat from the beef and slice into three-inch segments. Sprinkle with pepper and salt.

3. In a blender, puree the water, cloves, chipotles, oregano, lime juice, onion, garlic, and cumin. Pour in the oil, and brown the meat for about 5 minutes. Add the sauce (from the blender) and the bay leaves.

4. Cook for 65 minutes (sauté mode with the top on) until it's easily shredded with two forks. Add water if needed to ensure it remains moist.

5. When ready, arrange on a serving platter, shred, and add it back to the pot. Save the juices for later and remove the bay leaves.

6. Measure 1.5 cups of the reserved juices, and put 1/2 of a teaspoon of cumin and salt.

7. Serve once it has warmed up and the flavors have blended.

37.   *BBQ Flank Steak*

Serving Yields Provided: 8

Macro Counts - Each Serving:

- Net Carbs: 1 g
- Total Fats: 21 g
- Protein: 35 g
- Calories: 342

Ingredients Needed:

- Flank steak (3 lb.)
- Paprika (1 tsp.)
- Granulated garlic (1 tsp.)
- Cayenne pepper (1 tsp.)
- Granulated onion (1 tsp.)
- White pepper (1 tsp.)
- Salt (1 tsp.)
- Black pepper (1 tsp.)
- Coconut aminos (1 tbsp.)
- Water (.25 cup)
- Melted butter (2 tbsp.)

Directions for Preparation:

1. Combine the aminos, seasonings, and melted butter. Rub into the steak.
2. Add the water to the cooker and the steak fixings.
3. Cook it for 8 hours, flipping halfway through the cooking cycle.
4. Serve with some creamy spinach.

38.   *Cheeseburger Calzones*

Serving Yields Provided: 8

Macro Counts - Each Serving:

- Net Carbs: 3 g
- Total Fats: 47 g
- Protein: 34 g
- Calories: 580

Ingredients Needed:

- Dill pickle spears (4)
- Cream cheese - divided (8 oz.)
- Shredded mozzarella cheese (1 cup)
- Egg (1)
- Almond flour (1 cup)
- Lean ground beef (1.5 lb.)
- Yellow diced onion (.5 of 1)
- Thick-cut bacon strips (4)
- Mayonnaise (.5 cup)
- Shredded cheddar cheese (1 cup)

Directions for Preparation:

1. Program the oven to 425° Fahrenheit.

2. Prepare a cookie tin with parchment paper.

3. Chop the pickles into spears. Set aside for now.

4. Prepare the crust. Combine half of the cream cheese and mozzarella cheese. Microwave for 35 seconds. When it melts, add the egg and almond flour to make the dough. Set aside.

5. Cook the beef on the stove using medium heat. Cook the bacon using the microwave or stovetop for 5 minutes. When it has cooled, break it into bits.

6. Dice the onion and add to the beef. Cook it until softened. Toss in the bacon, cheddar cheese, pickle bits, the rest of the cream cheese, and mayonnaise. Stir well.

7. Roll the dough onto the prepared baking tin. Scoop the mixture into the center. Fold the ends and sides to make the calzone.

8. Bake it until browned or for about 15 minutes. Let it rest for 10 minutes before slicing.

39.   *Enchilada*

Serving Yields Provided: 4

Macro Counts - Each Serving:

- Net Carbs: 7 g
- Total Fats: 30 g
- Protein: 36 g
- Calories: 455

Ingredients Needed:

- Small yellow onion (1)
- Ground beef (1.5 lb.)
- Red enchilada sauce (.66 cup)
- Chopped green onions (8)
- Diced Roma tomatoes (2)
- Shredded cheddar cheese (4 oz.)
- *Optional*: Freshly chopped cilantro (as desired)

Directions for Preparation:

1. Use a wok or skillet to sauté the yellow onion and meat.
2. Drain the juices and fold in the green onions, tomato, and enchilada sauce.

3. Once it starts to boil, simmer for about 5 minutes. Sprinkle with salt and cheese. Continue cooking until the cheese has melted.

4. Stir in the cilantro. Serve over chopped lettuce and a serving of sour cream. Add the extra carbs and enjoy.

INTERMITTENT
FASTING

CHAPTER 6:

Snacktime Treats

40.   *Arancini – 5-Cheese Bacon & Cauliflower Bites*

Serving Yields Provided: 10, 3 balls each
Macro Counts - Each Serving:

- Net Carbs: 5.4 g
- Total Fats: 19 g
- Protein: 19 g
- Calories: 280

Ingredients Needed:

- Riced cauliflower (5 cups)
- Bacon (1 lb.)
- Cream cheese (8 oz.)
- Goat cheese (4 oz.)
- Sharp cheddar cheese (.5 cup)
- Grated parmesan cheese (1.5 cups, divided)
- Sharp garlic & white cheddar cheese (.5 cup)
- Garlic (3 cloves)
- Italian seasoning, divided (1 tsp.)

- Black pepper (.5 tsp.)
- Onion powder (1 tsp.)
- Garlic powder (1 tsp.)
- Crushed pork rinds (1 cup)
- Panko or extra crushed pork rinds (.5 cup)
- Sea salt (.5 tsp.)
- Oil (as needed)

Directions for Preparation:

1. Cook and crumble the bacon. Let the cream cheese sit out a few minutes to soften. Prepare the cauliflower. Pulse it in a food processor or cheese grater. Mince the garlic and crush the pork rinds.

2. Combine the bacon, riced cauliflower, goat cheese, softened cream cheese, sharp cheddar cheese, .5 tsp Italian seasoning, sharp garlic, and white cheddar cheese, .5 cup grated Parmesan, minced garlic, sea salt, and pepper.

3. Combine all of the fixings until incorporated well. Refrigerate for 1 to 2 hours until it's firm.

4. Mix the crushed pork rinds, the rest of the parmesan cheese, panko, the rest of the Italian seasoning, onion powder, and garlic powder for the breading.

5. After the cauliflower mixture has chilled and is firm, roll the mixture into balls. Freeze for 3 hours or overnight.

6. Pour oil, measuring 1-inch thick, and heat it using the medium-high temperature setting.

7. Roll each of the balls in the breading mixture until all balls are evenly coated.

8. When the oil is hot, drop the balls into the pan, and fry the balls, five or six at a time. Fry them until they are evenly browned to your liking.

9. Transfer to a paper-lined platter. Serve.

41.   *BBQ Chicken Pizza*

Serving Yields Provided: 4

Macro Counts - Each Serving:

- Net Carbs: 6.5 g
- Total Fats: 16 g
- Protein: 24 g
- Calories: 282

Ingredients Needed:

- Parmesan cheese (3 oz.)
- Psyllium husk powder (3 tbsp.)
- Pepper & salt (1-2 pinches)
- Large eggs (6)
- Italian seasoning (1.5 tsp.)
- Shredded chicken (6 oz.)
- Barbecue sauce (4 tbsp.)
- Cheddar cheese (4 oz.)
- Tomato sauce (4 tbsp.)
- Mayonnaise (1 tbsp.)

Directions for Preparation:

1. Heat the oven until it reaches 425° Fahrenheit.

2. Shred the cheese. Combine the psyllium powder, parmesan, eggs, pepper, salt, and Italian seasoning. Once the dough has thickened, arrange it on a parchment paper to fit on a baking tin.

3. Bake it on the top rack of the oven for 10 minutes. Flip the crust, and add the rest of the fixings. Broil on high for 3 minutes and serve.

4. The total time to cook the pizza from start to finish is just 20 minutes.

42.   *Chicken Nuggets*

Serving Yields Provided: 6

Macro Counts - Each Serving:

- Net Carbs: 2 g
- Total Fats: 17 g
- Protein: 18 g
- Calories: 243

Ingredients Needed:

- Cooked chicken (2 cups)
- Cream cheese (8 oz.)
- Egg (1)
- Garlic salt (1 tsp.)
- Almond flour (.25 cup)

Directions for Preparation:

1. Set the oven temperature to 350° Fahrenheit.
2. Lightly grease a baking pan with a spritz of cooking oil spray. You can also use a layer of parchment paper.
3. Shred the chicken using a food processor or by hand. (Try using a combination of dark and light meat.)
4. Combine the rest of the fixings and mix well.

5. Scoop the nugget mixture onto the baking tin.
6. Bake it until firm and slightly browned (12 to 14 min.).

43.   *Chicken Salad Deviled Eggs*

Serving Yields Provided: 6

Macro Counts - Each Serving:

- Net Carbs: 2 g
- Total Fats: 7 g
- Protein: 13 g
- Calories: 128

Ingredients Needed:

- Old Bay Seasoning (1 dash)
- Lemon pepper (.5 tsp.)
- Dill (.5 tsp.)
- Celery salt (1 pinch)
- Chopped onion (1 tbsp.)
- Dijon mustard (1 tsp.)
- Mayonnaise (2 tbsp.)
- Shredded chicken (1 cup)
- Eggs (6 large)

Directions for Preparation:

1. Combine all of the fixings, and omit the eggs. Store it in the fridge for later.

2. Gently place the eggs in a pot of water (just enough to cover the eggs).

3. Set the temperature on high until it boils, and then lower the setting to medium.

4. Boil for 15 minutes and transfer to cool under cold running water.

5. Remove the shell, and slice the eggs into halves. Remove the yolk and fill with the salad mixture. Sprinkle with the old bay seasoning.

6. *Note*: Discard the yolks or use in another recipe. Total time is just 30 minutes.

44. *Delicious Grilled Cheese Sandwiches*

Serving Yields Provided: 2

Macro Counts - Each Serving:

- Net Carbs: 5 g
- Total Fats: 46 g
- Protein: 116 g
- Calories: 520

Ingredients Needed:

- Unsalted butter, divided (5 tbsp.)
- Whole milk, divided (4 tbsp.)
- Eggs, divided (2 large)
- Salt, divided (.25 tsp.)
- Coconut flour, divided (4 tbsp.)
- Baking powder, divided (1 tsp.)
- Sharp cheddar (2 oz.)

Directions for Preparation:

1. Add 2 tablespoons of butter into the dish. Microwave for about 50 seconds or until melted.
2. Mix in 2 tbsp of milk, 1 egg, and 1/8 tsp salt.

3. Add 2 tbsp coconut flour and 1/2 tsp baking powder. Mix until thoroughly combined.
4. Microwave the butter for 90 seconds. Allow it to rest for a minute.
5. Loosen the edges of the bread from the container. Arrange the bread on a rack to cool. Repeat the steps to make a second slice of keto bread.
6. Warm 1 tablespoon of butter in a skillet using the medium-low temperature setting.
7. Assemble the sandwich by placing two cheese slices between the keto bread slices you just made.
8. Once the butter foams, place the sandwich in the skillet.
9. Bake until the cheese has melted or 3 to 5 minutes on each side using medium-low heat.
10. Press on the sandwich with a large spatula.
11. Put the keto grilled cheese sandwich on a platter, and slice it into two triangles and serve.

Sweet Snacks

45.   *Cinnamon Vanilla Protein Bites*

Serving Yields Provided: 18–20 bites

Macro Counts - Each Serving:
- Net Carbs: 4 g
- Total Fats: 9 g
- Protein: 2 g
- Calories: 112

Ingredients Needed:
- Quick oats (.75 cup)
- Nut butter of choice (.25–.33 cup)
- Cinnamon (1 tbsp.)
- Pure maple syrup (.25–.33 cup)
- Vanilla protein powder (.25 cup)
- Almond meal (.5 cup)
- Vanilla extract (.5–1 tsp.)
- *Also Needed:* Food processor

Directions for Preparation:

1. Line a cookie tin with a layer of parchment paper.
2. Grind the oats with the processor and add to a mixing container. Combine the cinnamon, protein powder, almond meal, and nut butter.
3. Mix in the syrup and vanilla. Using your hands, mix and roll them into small balls.
4. Freeze for 20 to 30 minutes.
5. Store in a Ziploc-type bag with the cinnamon and vanilla protein mixture.

CHAPTER 7:

Dessert Favorites

46.   *Almond & Coconut Cake*

Serving Yields Provided: 8

Macro Counts - Each Serving:

- Net Carbs: 3 g
- Total Fats: 23g
- Protein: 5 g
- Calories: 236

Dry Ingredients Needed:

- Almond flour (1 cup)
- Truvia (.33 cup)
- Baking powder (1 tsp.)
- Unsweetened shredded coconut (.5 cup)
- Apple pie spice (1 tsp.)

Wet Ingredients Needed:

- Melted butter (.25 cup)

- Lightly whisked eggs (2)
- Heavy whipping cream (.5 cup)

Directions for Preparation:

1. Combine all of the dry ingredients, and add each of the wet ingredients, one at a time. Empty the batter into the pan, and cover with foil.
2. Empty the water into the Kitchen robot, and place the steamer rack inside.
3. Set the timer 40 minutes using the high-pressure setting. Release the pressure naturally for 10 minutes, and then quick-release it.
4. Remove the pan, and let it cool for 15 to 20 minutes.
5. Flip it over onto a platter and garnish as desired (count the carbs).
6. It is very important to cool the cake completely before you add the toppings.

47.   *Brownie Mug Cake – Kitchen robot*

Serving Yields Provided: 1

Macro Counts - Each Serving:

- Net Carbs: 1.3 g
- Protein: 9 g
- Total Fats: 12 g
- Calories: 143

Ingredients Needed:

- Whisked egg (1)
- Almond flour (.25 cup)
- Baking powder (.25 tsp.)
- Vanilla extract (.25 tsp.)
- Cacao powder (1.5 tbsp.)
- Cinnamon powder (1 tsp.)
- Stevia powder (2 tbsp.)
- Salt (1 pinch)

Directions for Preparation:

1. Pour one cup of water and the trivet or steam rack into the Kitchen robot.
2. Mix all of the fixings until well-combined, and pour it into a mug.

3. Cover with a piece of foil and place on the rack.

4. Secure the top.

5. Set the timer for 10 minutes using the "steam" button. Naturally, release the pressure (10 min.).

6. Cool for a minute and enjoy.

48.   *Cheesecake Pudding*

Serving Yields Provided: 4

Macro Counts - Each Serving:

- Net Carbs: 5 g
- Total Fats: 36 g
- Protein: 5 g
- Calories: 356

Ingredients Needed:

- Cream cheese or Neufchatel cheese (1 block)
- Heavy whipping cream (.5 cup)
- Lemon juice (1 tsp.)
- Sour cream (.5 cup)
- Liquid stevia (20 drops)
- Vanilla extract (1 tsp.)

Directions for Preparation:

1. Microwave the cream cheese for 30 seconds, or leave it on the counter to soften for a few minutes before using.
2. Whip the sour cream and whipping cream together with the mixer until soft peaks form. Combine with the rest of the fixings and whip until fluffy.

3. Portion it into four dishes to chill. Place a layer of the wrap over the dish and store in the fridge.
4. When ready to eat, garnish with some berries if you like. If you add berries, make sure to add the carbs to the count.

49.   *Chocolate Chip Cookie Cheesecake Bars*

Serving Yields Provided: 20

Macro Counts - Each Serving:

- Net Carbs: 5 g
- Protein: 5 g
- Total Fats: 25 g
- Calories: 280

Ingredients Needed - Cookies Crust:

- Almond flour (2 cups)
- Shredded coconut (1 cup)
- Salt (.25 tsp.)
- Swerve Sweetener (.5 cup)
- Baking powder (1.5 tsp.)
- Softened butter (.5 cup)
- Coconut sugar or more Swerve (2 tbsp.)
- Room temperature egg (1 large)
- Vanilla extract (.75 tsp.)
- Sugar-free chocolate chips (.5 cup)

Ingredients Needed - Cheesecake Filling:

- Large egg (1)
- Cream cheese, softened (12 oz.)
- Powdered swerve (.33 cup)
- Whipping cream (.25 cup)
- Vanilla extract (.5 tsp.)
- *Also Needed*: 9-inch square baking pan

Directions for Preparation - The Crust:

1. Warm the oven to 325° Fahrenheit.
2. Generously grease the pan.
3. Whisk the baking powder with the shredded coconut, almond flour, and salt in the mixing bowl.
4. In another container, beat the swerve with butter and coconut sugar. Whisk the vanilla and egg. Combine it with the flour mixture, and stir in the chocolate chips.
5. Press about 2/3 of the crust dough into the greased pan.
6. Bake for 10 to 12 minutes.
7. Take the tray out of the oven. Cool before adding the filling.

Directions for Preparation - The Filling:

1. Use a wooden spoon to blend the cheese with the sweetener and whipping cream until combined.

2. Whisk the vanilla extract and egg until smooth. Pour over the cooled crust.

3. Use the remainder of the cookie crust mixture to crumble over the top of the filling. Press gently to adhere.

4. Bake until the crust is nicely browned or for about 25 minutes. It will have just a little "jiggle" in the center.

5. Transfer from the oven to cool completely.

6. Chill for at least 1 hour until set.

50. *Chocolate-Filled Peanut Butter Cookies*

Serving Yields Provided: 20

Macro Counts - Each Serving:

- Net Carbs: 2.7 g
- Protein: 4.5 g
- Total Fats: 14 g
- Calories: 150

Ingredients Needed:

- Almond flour (2.5 cups)
- Baking powder (1.5 tsp.)
- Salt (.5 tsp.)
- Peanut butter (.5 cup)
- Coconut oil (.25 cup)
- Erythritol (.25 cup)
- Maple syrup (3 tbsp.)
- Dark chocolate bars (2-3)
- Vanilla extract (1 tbsp.)

Directions for Preparation:

1. Prepare the cookie pan with a baking paper.
2. Warm the oven to reach 350° Fahrenheit.

3. Whisk each of the wet fixings together and mix with the dry ingredients.
4. Mix well and store in the refrigerator for 20 to 30 minutes.
5. Break the bars into small squares. Press them until they are flat.
6. Add one to two pieces of chocolate and seal them into the ball.
7. Arrange them on the cookie sheet.
8. Bake for about 15 minutes.

51.   _Chocolate Mini Cakes_

Serving Yields Provided: 2

Macro Counts - Each Serving:

- Net Carbs: 9 g
- Total Fats: 12 g
- Protein: 15 g
- Calories: 193

Ingredients Needed:

- Large eggs (2)
- Splenda/your favorite sweetener (2 tbsp.)
- Baking cocoa (.25 cup)
- Heavy cream (2 tbsp.)
- Baking powder (.5 tsp.)
- Vanilla extract (1 tsp.)
- Water (1 cup)

Directions for Preparation:

1. Add the water and trivet into the Kitchen robot.
2. Combine all of the dry ingredients and mix well.
3. Mix in another dish, and blend in the rest of the ingredients (eggs, cream, vanilla extract).

4. Spray the ramekins with oil, and fill each one halfway with the mixture. Carefully add them to the cooker and secure the lid.

5. Prepare for 9 minutes using the high-pressure setting.

6. Quick-release the pressure, and transfer the ramekins to a plate to cool.

7. Make sure they are cool before adding toppings, or you can serve hot right out of the ramekins.

52. *Coconut-Almond Bars – Kitchen robot*

Serving Yields Provided: 6

Macro Counts - Each Serving:

- Net Carbs: 2 g
- Total Fats: 25 g
- Protein: 5 g
- Calories: 253

Ingredients Needed:

- Coconut oil (.5 cup)
- Almond flour (1.25 cups)
- Coconut flour (.25 cup
- Eggs (2)
- Sugar substitute (3 tbsp.)
- Almond butter (2 tbsp.)
- Salt (.25 tsp.)
- Water (1 cup)
- Vanilla extract (1 tsp.)

Also Needed:

- Trivet for the Cooker & Baking pan to fit inside
- Food processor

Directions for Preparation:

1. Line the pan that fits in the cooker with the baking paper.
2. Combine all of the fixings in the food processor and add to the pan.
3. Empty the water into the Kitchen robot with the steamer rack. Arrange the pan in the cooker and secure the lid.
4. Set the timer for 15 minutes.
5. Natural-release the pressure and chill the pan until its room temperature.
6. Slice into six bars.

53.   *Creamy Lime Pie*

Serving Yields Provided: 8

Macro Counts - Each Serving:

- Net Carbs: 4.2 g
- Protein: 7 g
- Total Fats: 38.6 g
- Calories: 386

Ingredients Needed:

- Almond flour (1.5 cups)
- Erythritol (divided, .5 cup)
- Salt (.5 tsp.)
- Melted butter (.25 cup)
- Heavy cream (1 cup)
- Egg yolks (4)
- Freshly squeezed key lime juice (.33 cup)
- Lime zest (1 tbsp.)
- Cubed cold butter (.25 cup)
- Vanilla extract (1 tsp.)
- Xanthan gum (.25 tsp.)
- Sour cream (1 cup)
- Cream cheese (.5 cup)

Directions for Preparation:

1. Warm the oven to 350° Fahrenheit.

2. Melt the butter in a pan.

3. Mix the salt, half or .25 cup of erythritol, and the almond flour. Slowly add the butter. Blend and press into a pie platter.

4. Bake for 15 minutes. Remove when it's lightly browned. Let it cool.

5. In another saucepan, combine the egg yolks, heavy cream, and the rest of the erythritol, lime zest, and juice.

6. Simmer using medium heat for 7 to 10 minutes or until it starts to thicken.

7. Take the pan from the heat, and add the xanthan gum, vanilla extract, cold butter, cream cheese, and sour cream. Whisk until smooth.

8. Scoop into the cooled pie shell. Cover and place in the fridge.

9. You can serve after 4 hours, but it is better if you wait overnight to enjoy the delicious treat.

54.   *5-Minute Peanut Butter Mousse*

Serving Yields Provided: 4

Macro Counts - Each Serving:

- Net Carbs: 3 g
- Total Fats: 26.5 g
- Protein: 5.9 g
- Calories: 301

Ingredients Needed:

- Heavy whipping cream, more if needed to thin the mixture (.5 cup)
- Cream cheese, softened (4 oz.)
- Natural peanut butter, no sugar added (.25 cup)
- Powdered Swerve Sweetener (.25 cup)
- Vanilla extract (.5 tsp.)

Directions for Preparation:

1. Whisk or whip the cream until it holds stiff peaks. Set aside.
2. In another medium bowl, beat together the cream cheese and peanut butter until smooth and creamy. Add the sweetener and vanilla. If your peanut butter is unsalted, add a pinch of salt as well. Beat until smooth.

3. If your mixture is very thick, add about 2 tbsp heavy cream to lighten it. Beat it again until combined.

4. Gently fold in the whipped cream until no streaks remain. Spoon or pipe into dessert glasses.

55.   _Keto Magic Bars_

Serving Yields Provided: 16

Macro Counts - Each Serving:

- Net Carbs: 4.5 g
- Total Fats: 12.4 g
- Protein: 1.8 g
- Calories: 132

Ingredients Needed:

- Almond flour (1.5 cups)
- Sweetener of choice, or stevia equivalent (2 tbsp.)
- Melted coconut oil (3 tbsp.)
- Salt (.25 tsp.)
- Mini chocolate chips or sugar-free chocolate chips (.75 cup)
- Full-fat shredded coconut (.66 cup)
- Full-fat canned coconut milk (1.25 cup)
- _Optional:_ Walnuts (.25 cup)
- _Optional_: Cocoa powder (2 tbsp.)
- _Also Needed_: 8-inch baking pan

Directions for Preparation:

1. Finely chop the walnuts. Prepare the pan with a layer of parchment baking paper.

2. Toss the salt, sweetener, almond flour, and oil together in the mixing bowl.

3. Press the mixture into the papered pan.

4. Toss the coconut, chips of chocolate, and nuts over the top.

5. Stir the cocoa with the coconut milk. Pour this evenly over the top.

6. Bake for 33 minutes.

7. Transfer the bars from the oven.

8. Let them cool for about 15 minutes to firm up.

9. Slice into bars, wiping the knife after each cut.

CHAPTER 8:

21-Day Special Meal Plan for Busy People

Each of these recipes has the net carbs per serving posted. You will see how flexible the plan is when you look at how easy it is to use the recipes in this cookbook for 21 full days, including three meals, snacks, and desserts.

The meals are planned, so you still have flexibility in your eating patterns with extra carbs to use as desired. Even on the strictest diet plan, most of these recipes should be just what the doctor ordered. You have plenty of extra choices, so just enjoy.

Calculate how many carbs you are allowed each day, and add some healthy snacks or sides to the carb count. It's all up to you; just track everything.

Day 1:

Breakfast: Blueberry Flaxseed Muffins: 8.78 grams

Lunch: Egg Salad: 1.4 grams

Dinner: Mongolian Beef: 1.99 grams

Snack or Dessert: Stuffed Mushrooms: 3 grams

Day 2:

Breakfast: Eggs & Sausage Breakfast Sandwich: 6 grams

Lunch: Jalapeno Popper Chicken Salad: 0 grams

Dinner: Stuffed Pork Tenderloin on the Grill: 3 grams

Snack or Dessert: Creamy Lime Pie: 4.2 grams

Day 3:

Breakfast: Pulled Pork Hash: 8 grams

Lunch: Simple Red Cabbage Salad: 0.2 grams

Dinner: BBQ Flank Steak: 1 gram

Snack or Dessert: Pumpkin Caramel Bundt Cake: 5 grams

Day 4:

Breakfast: Smoothie in a Bowl: 4 grams

Lunch: Sloppy Joes – Vegan: 8.9 grams

Dinner: Chicken BBQ Zucchini Boats: 9 grams

Snack or Dessert: Vanilla Shortbread Cookies: 1 gram

Day 5:

Breakfast: Green Buttered Eggs: 2.5 grams

Lunch: Chicken BLT Salad: 4 grams

Dinner: Hamburger Stroganoff: 6 grams

Snack or Dessert: Chocolate Chip Cookie Cheesecake Bars:
5 grams

Day 6:

Breakfast: Cinnamon Raisin Bagels: 6 grams

Lunch: Chicken 'Zoodle' Soup: 4 grams

Dinner: Carnitas – Crockpot: 4 grams

Snack or Dessert: Peanut Butter Fudge: 6 grams

Day 7:

Breakfast: Porridge: 5.4 grams

Lunch: Avocado & Salmon Omelet Wrap: 5.8 grams

Dinner: Barbacoa Beef – Kitchen robot: 2 grams

Snack or Dessert: Raspberry Ice Cream: 3 grams

Day 8:

Breakfast: Belgian Style Waffles: 3 grams

Lunch: Vegetarian Club Salad: 5 grams

Dinner: Baked Tilapia With Cherry Tomatoes: 4 grams

Snack or Dessert: Vanilla Sour Cream Cupcake: 2 grams

Day 9:

Breakfast: Creamy Basil Baked Sausage: 4 grams

Lunch: Warm Peach Scallops Salad: 7 grams

Dinner: Nacho Skillet Steak: 6 grams

Snack or Dessert: Brownie Mug Cake – Kitchen robot: 1.3 grams

Day 10:

Breakfast: Almond Coconut Egg Wraps: 3 grams

Lunch: Chicken Chowder – Crockpot: 7.5 grams

Dinner: Lemon Shrimp: 2.5 grams & Arancini – 5-Cheese Bacon & Cauliflower Bites: 5.4 grams

Snack or Dessert: Sugar-Free Fudgesicles: 1.6 grams

Day 11:

Breakfast: Biscuits & Gravy: 2 grams

Lunch: Greek Salad: 8 grams

Dinner: Cheeseburger Calzones: 3 grams

Snack or Dessert: Keto Magic Bars: 4.5 grams

Day 12:

Breakfast: Pesto Scrambled Eggs: 2.6 grams

Lunch: Alfredo Shrimp: 6.5 grams

Dinner: Chicken & Asparagus: 4 grams

Snack or Dessert: Cheesecake Pudding: 5 grams

Day 13:

Breakfast: Spinach Quiche: 0 grams

Lunch: Chicken, Feta, & Kiwi Salad: 13 grams

Dinner: Bacon Cheeseburger: 0.8 grams

Snack or Dessert: Raspberry Fudge: 4.4 grams

Day 14:

Breakfast: Keto Hot Cross Buns: 2.1 grams

Lunch: Caprese Salad: 4.6 grams

Dinner: Roasted Chicken & Tomatoes: 5 grams

Snack or Dessert: Zucchini Chocolate Cake: 7.4 grams

Day 15:

Breakfast: Almost McGriddle Casserole: 3 grams

Lunch: No-Cook Chilled Avocado & Mint Soup: 4 grams

Dinner: Enchilada: 7 grams

Snack or Dessert: 5-Minute Peanut Butter Mousse: 3 grams

Day 16:

Breakfast: Chocolate Loaf: 2.32 grams

Lunch: Jar Salad with Tempeh – Vegan: 4 grams

Dinner: Slow-Cooked Kalua Pork & Cabbage: 4 grams

Snack or Dessert: Chocolate-Filled Peanut Butter Cookies: 2.7 grams

Day 17:

Breakfast: Bacon Hash: 9 grams

Lunch: Creamy Chicken Soup: 2 grams

Dinner: Slow-Cooked London Broil: 2.5 grams

Snack or Dessert: Almond & Coconut Cake: 3 grams

Day 18:

Breakfast: Cocoa Waffles: 3.4 grams

Lunch: Lobster Salad: 2 grams

Dinner: Parmesan Crusted Pork Chops: 3 grams

Snack or Dessert: Coconut Almond Bars – Kitchen robot: 2 grams

Day 19:

Breakfast: Pumpkin Pancakes: 4 grams

Lunch: Broccoli Curry Soup: 4.8 grams

Dinner: Crack Slaw – Pork Egg Roll in a Bowl: 5.5 grams

Snack or Dessert: No-Bake Chocolate Fudge Haystacks: 1.5 grams

Day 20:

Breakfast: Almonds & Chips Breakfast Cereal: 3 grams

Lunch: Fish Cakes: 0.6 grams & Chinese Sauce Fried Rice: 4.3 grams

Dinner: Sesame Chicken Egg Roll in a Bowl: 3.3 grams

Snack or Dessert: Cinnamon Vanilla Protein Bites: 4 grams

Day 21:

Breakfast: Bagels & Cheese: 8 grams

Lunch: Tuna Salad & Chives: 1 gram

Dinner: BBQ Pork Loin: 3 grams

Snack or Dessert: Chocolate Mini Cakes: 9 grams

CHAPTER 9:
Tips & Tricks to Control Hunger
&
Avoid Mistakes

How to Maintain Fat Loss

Remain Consistent During Fasting: Regardless of the type of weight loss that you ultimately choose to pursue, it's essential to pick one and stick with it. Attempting an intermittent fast for a few days using the keto diet plan before switching to another program, such as the Paleo diet, before trying out a low-carb approach will only cause your body to become confused. It will hold on to every possible calorie until it figures out what the changes mean.

Remember, fasting regularly and consistently is the surest way to see any of its benefits. Only after your body has time to adjust to your new routine will it then be able to adapt appropriately. It can begin to increase the number of positive enzymes and neural pathways to maximize weight loss using this method.

Consider consistency of the "ace-in-the-hole" of proactive weight loss success.

Maintain Your Self-Control: Intermittent fasting only works if your body goes entirely without food for at least twelve hours; any caloric intake resets the cycle. As such, it is imperative to ensure that you maintain control of your bodily urges if you hope to see real results from this type of approach. Remember, fasting for at least twelve hours will only allow you to eat as you usually would or slightly more than an average meal. It doesn't give you free rein to eat everything in sight. Keeping your appetite in check is a strict requirement for success.

Maintain a Calorie Deficit: While this is true for any diet, it is even more true for intermittent fasting since it can be so easy to overeat in such a way that it negates any benefits you might have felt. Remember, you need to burn 3,500 calories on average weekly to lose one pound each week.

Avoid Junk Food: While intermittent fasting means that you will likely have a little extra caloric room in your diet for junk food if you so choose, trying to eat poorly while intermittent fasting will only lead to failure. While you may technically be able to spare the calories, spending the ones you do have on things that won't stick to your ribs for the long haul is a recipe for disaster. Focus on foods that are high in protein and healthy fats. You will feel full and energetic for more prolonged periods every time. You only have so much time you can eat each day, so make it count.

Take It Slow: If you have never gone more than a few hours without eating, then it's a good idea to start slowly. You can go hours without eating and then build up your tolerance from there. It is important to go slow, so if you experience lots of failures early on, it can be more challenging to convince your brain to get into a pro-fasting mindset in the long term. Once you begin to see real weight loss results, you will notice that it will become easier to persevere; all you have to do is make it to that point, and things will begin to fall into place.

Be Aware Of Your Body's Response: While you will want to monitor how your body is reacting to the intermittent fasting process as long as you are regularly withholding calories, this is especially important during the first month while your body is transitioning to a new way of receiving calories. While you may feel faint, lightheaded, shaky, irritable, angry, or weak for up to a month while fasting, symptoms that persist indefinitely are a sign that something ultimately isn't right. It is essential to be in touch with your body enough to know when it's time to consult a health care professional.

Drink Tons of Water: This doesn't mean merely stay hydrated, which is good advice, regardless. It means you should drink at least a gallon of water each day. It will help you feel full and also ensure your body continues processing toxins normally, even if it is holding onto all of its fat because of the transition that is occurring. This is a good exercise for most people anyway, as roughly 40 percent of adults are in a mild state of dehydration. If thirst remains untreated for long enough, it starts manifesting itself as hunger, so staying hydrated will keep you feeling full longer in two ways.

Plan On Staying Busy: While this is a good suggestion in general when it comes to the final few hours of your fast, it's especially important during your transition period. Having nothing to do but sit around for several hours until you can eat again is a sure way to put your untrained body into a situation where it can't help but fail. Don't let this happen to you. Just ensure your fast will break after a period of constant mental activity, and you will find those last few hours going by much faster.

Get More Sleep & Less Stress: If you are a victim of sleep deprivation, you will understand how stressful everyday life is, even before you begin a diet plan. You may believe it's too late for you, but it isn't. Your diet plan will work, but you may need to make a few other adjustments.

Chronic stress will increase your cortisol levels—the stress hormone. With that action, your hunger levels also rise. The result is that you eat more and put on weight. It's important to find ways to remove the stress, whether it is decluttering your home or taking a vacation.

Eliminate coffee or other forms of caffeine early in the afternoon, and don't consume alcohol for at least three hours before bedtime. Alcohol will also interfere with your quality of sleep, which is why you wake up feeling tired after an evening of nightclubs and boozing.

Recognize Your Cravings

Sugary Foods: Several things can trigger one's desire for sugar, but typically, phosphorous, and tryptophan are the culprits. Have some chicken, beef, lamb, liver, cheese, cauliflower, or broccoli.

Chocolate: The carbon, magnesium, and chromium levels are requesting a portion of spinach, nuts, and seeds, or some broccoli and cheese. It's important to make sure you keep a healthy count of sodium, potassium, and magnesium in your diet. It is suggested to consume a minimum of two teaspoons daily. However, if you crave chocolate, eat chocolate. You need to make sure you eat 75% or higher dark chocolate. Omit milk chocolate from the diet plan.

Fatty or Oily Foods: The levels of calcium and chloride need repair with some spinach, broccoli, cheese, or fish.

Carbs/Bread/Pasta: You need some nitrogen, which can be remedied by eating high-protein meat.

Eat Healthier Snacks During Your Eating Window

Stock your pantry with plenty of high-quality snacks that you can eat when your resistance is down. When you choose snack items, always be sure to select ones that are low in carbs, so your ketone levels will not be disrupted. If you have a busy lifestyle, pick some of the items in the following list, but always remember to count the carbs.

- *Pork Rinds:* Use these to replace chips and crackers. For example, try Pork Clouds, which has a higher quality but without a lot of the offensive oil content.

- *Pepperoni Slices:* Enjoy them with high-fat cheese products, but keep in mind that these are highly processed. Limit your intake of this, and search for hormone-free meat or organic food, if possible.

- *String Cheese:* Choose the full-fat version without additional fillers.

- *Laughing Cow Cheese Wheels:* Purchase full-fat versions and get *real* cheese when possible.

- *Iced Coffee*: Leave the sugar out of your coffee, and use only full-fat milk or cream. Add a bit of MCT oil powder, which can be purchased as chocolate, vanilla, or unflavored.

- *Stevia Sweetened Dark Chocolate*: If you are not using stevia, make sure it's a minimum of 80% or higher in cocoa content.

- *Cacao Nibs*: You can enjoy the same crunch when used as an alternative to chocolate chips.

- *Sugar-Free Jell-O or Popsicles*: You can purchase this ready-to-go, or you can make your own.

Be Sure the Plan Is for You—Avoid Mistakes

As with other things in your life, intermittent fasting may not be for you. You may need to avoid the restrictions if you are included in these categories:

- People with eating disorder histories

- If you are taking prescription medications, you can have issues on taking them on an empty stomach. If you have diabetes, Metformin may cause diarrhea or nausea. Iron supplements may also cause stomach discomfort. Aspirin may also cause an upset stomach or possible ulcers.

- Individuals with diabetes mellitus: type 1 or type 2

- Individuals who experience a drop in his/her blood sugar levels many times

- People who are underweight (BMI≤ 18.5), malnourished, or have other known nutrient deficiencies

- Pregnant women will need more nutrition for the unborn child.

- Nursing mothers will require more nutrients for the baby.

- Children under 18 need more nutrients to grow.

Other Intermittent Dieting Suggestions

If you have tried the 16/8 plan without success, try one of these options.

Skipping Meals: If you're interested in trying out the benefits of intermittent fasting for yourself, but you have an irregular schedule or are not sure if it is for you, then skipping a meal or two, now and then, maybe the type of intermittent fasting for you. As previously discussed, getting into a fasting routine is vital to see the maximum results for your effort, but that doesn't occasionally mean that fasting doesn't come with some benefits as well.

What's more, once you have tried skipping a meal now and then, you can see for yourself just how easy it is, which, in turn, can lead to more positive changes in the future. With so many intermittent fasting options available, the odds are good that one fits your schedule, so give it a try. What have you got to lose, except for a bunch of unessential pounds?

Alternate Day Diet: This form of intermittent fasting means you never have to go long without food if you don't wish to fast for an extended time. Every other day, you should eat regularly, and on the off-days, you merely consume one-fifth of the calories you usually intake on average days.

The average daily caloric consumption is between 2,000 and 2,500 calories, which means that the regular off-day varies between 400 and 500 calories. If you enjoy exercising every day, then this form of intermittent fasting may not be for you since you will have to limit your workouts on off-days severely.

When you first begin this technique of intermittent fasting, the easiest way to make it through the low-calorie days is by trying any the protein shakes listed. It is important to work back to "real" natural foods these days because they will always be healthier than the shakes.

This form of intermittent fasting is all about losing weight. Those who try it tend to average between two and three pounds lost per week. If you attempt the Alternate Day Diet, it is critical to eat regularly on your full-calorie days. Binging will not only negate any progress you've made, but it can also cause severe damage to your body if continued over time.

Crescendo Method: This is a method that is ranked as one method suitable for women since you can begin fasting without irritating your hormones or shocking any part of your body using this technique. This is one of the safest programs for women who utilize a fasting window of 12-16 hours. You can enjoy your meals for 8-12 hours. Space it out for a few days, such as Monday, Wednesday, and Friday. If you have failed other diets, this might be your answer. After a two-week period, add one more day of active fasting to your schedule.

Always Check Your Medications for Compatibility

It's important to inform your doctor about your weight loss program. He/she may prescribe some medicines that make you gain weight.

If you are taking insulin injections in high doses, your insulin can impede weight loss. By consuming fewer carbs, you are substantially reducing the requirement of insulin. Again, ask your healthcare professional before you make any changes.

If you are attempting to lose weight, be aware of other

probable medications causing weight gain:

- Oral contraceptives
- Antidepressants
- Epilepsy drugs
- Blood pressure medications
- Allergy medicines
- Antibiotics

Know-How: Test for Ketosis Activity

Maintaining ketosis is an individual process, and you need to be sure you are achieving your goals. The levels of beta-hydroxybutyrate, acetone, and acetoacetate can be measured in your urine, breath, and blood.

You can use a *"Ketonix"* meter to measure your breath. You breathe into the meter. The results will be provided by a special coded color that will flash to show your levels of ketosis at that time.

Measure the ketones with a blood ketone meter. All it takes is a small drop of blood on a testing strip inserted into the meter. This process has been researched as an excellent indicator of your current ketosis levels. Unfortunately, the testing strips are expensive.

Test your urine for acetoacetate. The strip is dipped into the urine, which will change the color of the strip. The various shades of purple and pink indicate the levels of ketones. The darker the color on the testing strip, the higher the level of ketones. The major benefit of this is that they are inexpensive. The most effective time to test is early in the morning, after a ketogenic diet dinner, the evening before testing.
You should use one or more of these methods to indicate whether you need to adjust your intake of foods to remain in ketosis.

When you fast, the hormones in your body will change. The keto plan is similar to this process. You could achieve ketosis in just a couple of days once you have used up all your stored glycogen. It can take a month, a week, or just a few days. It all depends on which type of plan you choose. Your protein and carbohydrate intake will determine the time.

Conclusion

I hope you enjoyed every segment of *Intermittent Fasting*, from the first page to the end, and I hope you can now achieve your goals in weight loss or whatever they may be.

The next step is to gather your essential shopping list and knowledge on the ketogenic diet to travel to the supermarket.

- Prepare the food list consisting of your favorite spices and other products to convert your pantry to keto.

- Begin using your new diet plan, remembering that you can adjust the menu plan using the carbohydrate limitations set for each day. Keep your intake of carbs low.

- Prepare a food journal, and familiarize yourself with an online app to remain in ketosis with ease. You have all of the tools to be successful, but you still need to understand how to test yourself to ensure that you are in ketosis. Your individual progress can be tested using several items to ensure you remain in a ketogenic state. They include testing your breath, blood, or urine.

There is no time like the present to gather your lists of goods needed to begin your ketogenic way of living. Begin with your food and preparation items, and before you know it, you will be stocking your freezer to the brim with all the delicious keto foods your body is craving.

If you find yourself feeling excessively hungry in the early morning hours, the first thing you should keep in mind is that much of this hunger is actually mental, rather than physical. After you have finished the transition, you should notice it much less often. With that being said, it's important to start each day by drinking a liter of water. If you still feel hungry, consider ending your previous day's meal with extra protein and healthy fats which should stick with you through the morning.

Above all, reward yourself. After you have started losing weight, it is important to have a bit of fun. However, you should make sure that it is not a food-related treat. Treat yourself to a massage, or buy a new pair of jeans to show off your loss. Take the family for a game of putt-putt or enjoy a special spa treatment. You deserve it.

While you are considering your reward, why not have a delicious cup of coffee?

This Bulletproof Coffee is for one serving with zero carbs. It has 51 total fats, 1 protein, and 320 calories.

Ingredients Needed:

- MCT oil powder (2 tbsp.)
- Ghee or butter (2 tbsp.)
- Hot coffee (1.5 cups)

Directions for Preparation:

1. Empty the hot coffee into your blender.
2. Pour in the powder and butter. Blend until frothy.
3. Enjoy using a large mug.

Finally, if you found this book useful in any way, a review on Amazon is always appreciated!

8 hrs

16 hrs

Index For The Recipes:

Chapter 3: Breakfast Favorites

1. Almond Coconut Egg Wraps
2. Almonds & Chips Breakfast Cereal
3. Almost McGriddle Casserole
4. Bacon Hash
5. Bagels & Cheese
6. Belgian Style Waffles
7. Biscuits & Gravy
8. Blueberry Flaxseed Muffins
9. Blueberry Ricotta Pancakes
10. Chocolate Loaf
11. Cinnamon Raisin Bagels
12. Classic Bacon & Eggs
13. Cocoa Waffles

Chapter 4: Lunchtime Options

1. Bread Twists for the Salad
2. Caprese Salad
3. Chicken BLT Salad
4. Chicken, Feta, & Kiwi Salad

5. Chicken-Pecan Salad & Cucumber Bites
6. Cobb Salad
7. Egg Salad
8. Greek Salad

Soup Choices

1. Broccoli Curry Soup
2. Chicken Chowder – Crockpot

Seafood

1. Alfredo Shrimp
2. Avocado & Salmon Omelet Wrap

Other Delicious Lunchtime Choices

1. Buffalo Cauliflower Bites
2. Chinese Sauce Fried Rice

Chapter 5: Tasty Dinner Choices

Poultry

1. Buffalo Chicken Burgers
2. Chicken & Asparagus

Pork Options

1. BBQ Pork Loin

2. Carnitas – Crockpot

3. Crack Slaw – Pork Egg Roll in a Bowl

Fish & Seafood Options

1. Baked Tilapia With Cherry Tomatoes

2. Chili Lime Cod

Beef Options

1. Bacon Cheeseburger

2. Barbacoa Beef – Kitchen robot

3. BBQ Flank Steak

4. Cheeseburger Calzones

5. Enchilada

Chapter 6: Snacktime Treats

1. Arancini – 5-Cheese Bacon & Cauliflower Bites

2. BBQ Chicken Pizza

3. Chicken Nuggets

4. Chicken Salad Deviled Eggs

5. Delicious Grilled Cheese Sandwiches

Sweet Snacks

1 Cinnamon Vanilla Protein Bites

Chapter 7: Dessert Favorites

1. Almond & Coconut Cake
2. Brownie Mug Cake – Kitchen robot
3. Cheesecake Pudding
4. Chocolate Chip Cookie Cheesecake Bars
5. Chocolate-Filled Peanut Butter Cookies
6. Chocolate Mini Cakes
7. Coconut Almond Bars – Kitchen robot
8. Creamy Lime Pie
9. 5-Minute Peanut Butter Mousse
10. Keto Magic Bars